408676

613.25
Dav

unque 14.95

W9-AVS-678

# Better Than Atkins

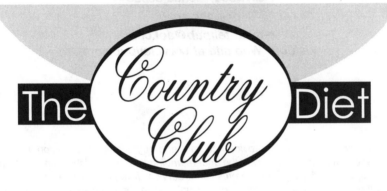

## The Country Club Diet

## America's Weight Solution

DISCARD

# By Debi Davis & Sylvan R. Lewis, M.D.

Shelbyville-Shelby County
Public Library

408676

## Frederick Fell Publishers, Inc.

2131 Hollywood Boulevard, Suite 305
Hollywood, Florida 33020
954-925-5242
**e-mail: fellpub@aol.com**
**Visit our Web site at www.fellpub.com**

This publication is designed to provide accurate and authoritative information in regard to the subject matter covered. It is sold with the understanding that the publisher is not engaged in rendering legal, accounting, or other professional service. If legal advice or other assistance is required, the services of a competent professional person should be sought. From A Declaration of Principles jointly adopted by a Committee of the American Bar Association and a Committee of Publishers.

### Library of Congress Cataloging-in-Publication Data

Davis, Debi.
  Better than Atkins : the country club diet / by Debi Davis & Sylvan R. Lewis.
    p. cm.
  Includes index.
  ISBN 0-88391-118-3 (alk. paper)
  1. Reducing diets. 2. Low-carbohydrate diet. I. Title.
RM222.2.D33 2004
613.2'5--dc22

                                        2004011408

# Better Than Atkins

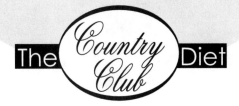

The Country Club Diet

## America's Weight Solution

*To every habitual & frustrated dieter...*
*your "weight" is over!*


*Enjoy the journey.*

# TABLE OF CONTENTS

# INTRODUCTION

I have been in the weight loss business with my partner and ex-husband, Byron, since 1991. During that time we have seen quite an evolution in the public's focus and direction on personal health and weight management. In 1991, most of our clients were unaware of the specifics associated with the food pyramid… didn't know a protein from a carbohydrate and had very little understanding of the term "holistic" when it came to medicine or healthcare. During the course of the last decade, we watched Americans embrace herbs like they were 'magic' solutions to their weight problems and use drugs like Lipitor as a means of protection against their continuing need to eat a diet rich in high cholesterol foods.

Americans have become smarter, but also more overweight than in any other time in history. We have more 'remedies' against poor health yet diabetes, heart disease, cancer and many other debilitating conditions are at an all time high. Our children are getting heart disease before they reach 30 years of age and just about every person we know has a friend or loved one currently fighting some fatal or debilitating disease. Why is that?

For more than a year following the 9-11 tragedy, Americans were eating comfort foods in abundance. With war pending, weight management was not in the forefront of America's mind and the result that followed was a much heavier and unhealthier population. In addition, people were taking more prescription drugs than any other time in our ten-plus year experience. As a company, our challenges had changed.

Byron and I understand the importance of addressing the human condition from a medical perspective and we enlisted the assistance of Dr. Sylvan. Lewis. Dr. Lewis is Board Certified in Internal Medicine and Cardiovascular Diseases and has a doctorate in Integrative Medicine. He was Health and Nutrition Advisor to the U.S. Department of Health, Education and Welfare and Chief of Cardiology at the U.S. Public Health Service Hospital in New Orleans, LA. Dr. Lewis provided us with first-hand knowledge of the effect food has on health as it relates to the body. He was quick to tell us 'food is a drug' and made it abundantly clear that nobody can lose weight when their body won't let them. As we dove more deeply into the subject, we saw from practical application how true Dr. Lewis' statement was.

My previous books and experience with weight management were predominantly treating the public's symptoms of overweight. With Dr. Lewis' help, I came to recognize that I was not adequately addressing the cause of my client's weight challenges. I've watched thousands of people struggle to get close to their goal while exercising fiendishly and eating the right foods, all with minimum success. What has happened to America that Americans remain the fattest people on the planet?

To create this work, we became a team; Byron, Dr. Lewis and myself. Dr. Lewis brings the medical expertise, Byron contributes nutritional research and I add the practical, yet confrontational perspective of the American public. Having personally lost 85 pounds in 1991 and keeping it off all these years, I know what the general population is or is not willing to do when it comes to health, nutrition and the maintenance of proper weight. But, once I learned how my body worked, it has been easy to make the changes that I never thought possible. I had been killing myself with the food I was eating. It's amazing how motivational the concept of 'shortened mortality' can have on a person!

Dr. Lewis has provided a simple understanding of the human condition from a physical perspective. Our 7-Day Hormone Diet is a revolutionary and scientific approach to an age-old problem that has frustrated and complicated the health of millions. Understanding this dietary model and utilizing its practical application for day-to-day life helped me make many necessary changes. As a result, I look better, feel better, am healthier and have more energy than I have had in years. I hope, after reading this along with a little personal reflection and application, you can say the same.

Enjoy!

Debi

# UNDERSTANDING THE CHALLENGE

Working on this project opened my eyes to a number of physical factors that I had been completely ignorant of for the last ten years. Weight management all boils down to this:

> **There are two types of people in the world: Thin People and Overweight People.**
> **Thin people are 'fat burners'.**
> **Overweight people are 'sugar burners'.**

The factor that determines which kind of person you are is your body's hormonal make-up. Your hormones are extremely powerful and essentially control most functions in your body. They are interconnected and work together to fine tune metabolism and other processes which regulate fat-burning ability. For example, insulin hormone regulates the body's sugar levels. Ghrelin hormone is produced in the stomach and intestine and controls hunger. Insulin regulates ghrelin concentration. These, along with other hormones like thyroid, estrogen, leptin (considered the 'obesity hormone'), growth hormone and many others must be balanced and harmonious in order for your body to be healthy and lean.

'Fat burners' have healthy hormones that are adequately balanced to provide them with tremendous energy reserves in their body for efficient metabolism. They rarely have weight problems. Their body tends to preserve and promote muscle growth and burns fat as fuel.

'Sugar burners' over-produce insulin hormone which causes the body to crave more. Whenever you stop eating and adequate amounts of sugar are not present, the body begins to cannibalize itself, eating muscle to make more sugar which ultimately turns into fat and increases body fat storage. Unless you help your body lower its sugar-insulin requirement, you are destined to be a 'sugar burner' with a weight challenge.

The connection between hormone health and its association with weight problems began during a lunchtime conversation where we were discussing the substantial increase in health challenges amongst our friends. Each of us were lamenting the fact that we all had friends and family members who had either just died from a heart attack, succumbed to their battle with cancer or developed diabetes. In all cases, the people we were discussing were under 55 years of age and one as young as 42. We began to question if people today really ARE living longer, or are we just being kept alive with drugs and medical procedures? The medical profession treats the symptoms of our diseases, but does it ever take the time to get to the cause?

Dr. Lewis has told Byron and me story after story of patients that he saw for heart disease who continued to maintain the same diet that initially created their clogged arteries and poor health condition. In many cases, the disease won and a heart attack or coronary bypass was its proof. Just about every doctor in America will tell you that the success of their practice is greatly compromised by the overall obesity of their patients. With over 66% of Americans overweight, is it no wonder that health disorders have never been higher?

To assume that there is no connection between the food we eat and the health we enjoy is nonsensical. The fact is, we ARE what we eat. I have asked myself why it is that just about anyone who drives a car, even those most ignorant of the car's mechanics, all know that they must put the right fuel in their vehicle in order for it to run properly. We know that leaded fuel in an unleaded fueled car will raise havoc on the engine. Then why is it so difficult to recognize that the fuel we put into our body can be just as dangerous and damaging as the wrong gasoline is to our automobile?

I truly believe people want to be healthier. They simply don't know what to do. For the most part, nobody likes change and diets can be overwhelming, complicated, and very inconvenient. Likewise, we all act like we understand what our 'hormones' do. Unfortunately, we connect raging ones with adolescent teens, PMS with cranky mates, hot flashes as part of the vestiges of aging and insulin with diabetes; all of which are somewhat accurate but hardly complete. You can control your weight, and your susceptibility to disease when you control your food intake because food chemistry controls your hormones.

Dr. Atkins was brilliant in his recognition of the association between insulin hormone and its effect on weight. He had his followers practically eliminate carbohydrates and, by doing so, he was altering their insulin production. At the same time, Dr. Atkins' required increase in protein consumption helped the body retain muscle mass, getting the patient closer to being a 'fat burner', not a 'sugar burner'. Unfortunately, even though the doctor's concept was very sound medically, practically speaking, it was almost impossible to follow for any length of time. In 2003, the New England Journal of Medicine reported more than a 40% dropout rate within six months of those starting the Atkins Diet. Within one year, there was no significant weight loss difference between the Atkins group and any other diet program.

Although the Atkins Diet is an effective means for short-term weight loss, the Atkins follower has not historically achieved long-term maintenance of their lost weight. People complain about the carbohydrate limitations although fruits and vegetables have been added back onto the diet over the years. In addition, irritability, fatigue as well as bowel, kidney and liver problems have all resulted from this well-meaning, but generally imbalanced program.

A large part of the medical complications Atkins' followers experience is due to the high fat content allowable on his program. Because you are able to eat fat in the forms of butter, cheese, heavy cream, pastrami and other high-fat meats, the high amount of fat, especially saturated fat in these items, has led to tremendous cholesterol elevation in some people. These fats also produce ketones in the urine which further explains the liver and kidney complication that so often affects Atkins dieters. Ketosis causes the loss of precious minerals in the urine that creates high acid levels and is not healthy for many reasons. The most critical reason is that when a large amount of acid is dumped into the blood, it interferes with the efficiency of thousands of reactions. When the blood has high-acid levels, red blood cells hold onto oxygen and cannot deliver it throughout the body. In this state, a person may feel fatigued or light headed. A hormonally balanced body is not acidic.

It is unfortunate that most doctors, including endocrinologists, do not understand that because our hormones are interconnected, they directly affect the levels of each other and food is the trigger. A diet high in sugar and carbohydrates increases insulin which, in turn, will decrease growth hormone and testosterone. Severe health and medical issues occur from decreasing these hormones which cause other hormonal imbalances in the body. The point is, food affects all hormones, often in a profound manner.

That stops now. This book will help you understand how your body works, why your hormones are a major factor in managing your weight and what role food plays in your overall health. We are not going to suggest you eat foods that, although they may be part of America's favorites, clearly make no sense from a health perspective. Let's face it, you can't eat unlimited fat and be fat free. The Country Club Diet is not 'magical'. It is a practical, safe and healthful, medically approved approach to fat loss and weight management.

## BREAKING THE METABOLIC FAT CYCLE

Your inability to affectively lose unwanted pounds and inches, up until now, may stem from a number of sources. Nutritional deficiencies and imbalances promote the storage of body fat which creates a "Metabolic Fat Cycle". When the body is undernourished, malnourished or suffers from chronic vitamin and mineral deficiencies, it will automatically slow its nutritional metabolic functions to conserve all sources of energy. In a rather abstract fashion, the metabolism slows as a protection method to keep the body from starving to death. This process causes the body to store more fat.

Body fat storage may stem from many factors including poor meal choices, pharmaceutical drug interactions, hereditary factors, and lifestyle. Your Metabolic Fat Cycle goes something like this:

- ① As weight is gained, the metabolism slows
- ① A slower metabolism then conspires with your nutritional imbalances and deficiencies to encourage even more storage of fat.
- ① The inevitable weight gain, in turn, increases nutritional and nutrient demands.
- ① The resulting nutritional imbalances promote additional weight gain and so the cycle continues.

Balanced nutrition is fundamental to healthy metabolism, fat loss and weight management. The weight loss benefits of nutritional balance cannot be overstated. When your body is in balance, the tendency to rapidly gain back lost weight (yo-yo dieting) is all but eliminated and uncontrolled food urges or binging will gradually subside.

Pharmaceutical drugs can cause nutrient depletion either by preventing absorption, enhancing nutrient elimination, or both. The senior population is even more susceptible to drug-induced depletions because seniors are more likely to receive multiple drugs for a variety of chronic aliments. Some of the more common drugs known to cause vitamin deficiencies include cardiovascular agents, anti-diabetic agents, anti-lipemic agents, anti-hypertensives, non-steroidal anti- inflammatory agents (NSAIDs), sedatives, hypnotics and antibiotics.

Over supplementation can be even more damaging to your health than taking too little. A four year study by the Food Standards Agency (U.K.) released the following information that may surprise you: "Vitamin C in large quantities can lead to stomach pain and diarrhea. Vitamin A can increase risk of osteoporosis. Too much Vitamin D can cause constipation, nausea and backaches. Over supplementation of Vitamin E can cause easy bruising, and muscle weakness." Unless your supplement use is being medically supervised, it is recommended that you take a simple multi-vitamin rather than a large variety of single nutrients.

## YOU CAN'T LOSE WEIGHT WHEN YOUR BODY WON'T LET YOU

Only five out of one hundred Americans successfully lose weight and maintain the loss. Weight and fat loss is not about discipline and willpower. It's about eliminating deficiencies, balancing hormones and nutritionally preparing your body, every day, to be efficient. Any tendency to overeat or experience food cravings simply means that your body has an imbalance that it is demanding be addressed. Unfortunately, giving in to cravings when you are unaware of their source, only perpetuates and even increases them.

Hormones play a major role in obtaining and maintaining your weight goal. When your endocrine system, which is your body's internal system of organs and glands that produce hormones is out of balance, no amount of exercising or dieting will correct your weight problem. Only through eating proper foods can you correct these imbalances, making weight management much easier in the future.

**The hormones that most affect weight control are:**

**Insulin:** The 'sugar hormone' controls sugar levels and is the master hormone in your body. It is so powerful that your body has four hormones: glucagon, adrenaline, noradrenaline, and cortisone, just to counter-balance and manage its effects. Insulin is responsible for organizing how your body uses the sugars and starches obtained from the food you eat. It is your 'storage hormone'. When disrupted, starches and sugars are turned into fat rather than being burned as a fuel. Both sweets, like desserts and candy as well as starches like potato or bread affect insulin levels in the body. When insulin is out of balance, overweight, diabetes and other diseases are created.

**Glucagon:** This hormone is made by your pancreas when blood sugar drops. Its major function is to steady blood sugar so your brain always has an adequate supply. When sugar drops, glucagon will break down muscle and fat to convert them to sugar via the liver. The most important relationship for determining the shape, size and amount of fat in your body is the insulin/glucagon ratio.

**Thyroid:** Is a gland located in your neck that secretes hormones that affect your physical shape, weight and temperament. It controls metabolism and the rate your body burns fat. When thyroid function is depressed, it leads to fatigue and a slowing of the metabolism which further contributes to weight gain.

**Ghrelin:** Produced mainly by the stomach, Ghrelin is also produced in the intestines and kidneys and is considered to be your 'hunger hormone'. In thin people, this hormone is at its highest level just before a meal and shuts down as you eat. In overweight people, this hormone continues to produce throughout a meal and is still activated when the meal is done, leaving the person to still feel hungry even after adequate amounts of food are consumed.

**Leptin:** The 'obesity hormone' is thought the be the hormone that tells the brain to curb appetite after eating. This hormone plays an important role in appetite suppression.

**Growth Hormone:** Made by the pituitary gland, this is the major anti-aging hormone which starts to decrease dramatically by age forty. Growth hormone causes muscles to grow and breaks down fat. In studies where additional growth hormone was injected into middle-aged men, there was a 14% loss of body fat and an 8% increase in muscle mass. This is the ideal situation for health and weight loss. You can use foods, appropriate lifestyle and exercise to maximize growth hormone level. Growth hormone works synergistically with testosterone to promote a trim body.

**Cortisol:** Is the stress hormone made by the adrenal glands. It comes into play when blood sugar drops or when you experience severe stress. Its action is to break down muscle tissue which can then be converted into sugar. High cortisol levels created when the body is stressed also promotes fat accumulation, especially around the waist.

**Testosterone:** A hormone made by the testes and the adrenal glands in males, and in the adrenal glands in females. It encourages muscle growth, mass, strength and muscle maintenance in both sexes. Low levels of testosterone promote increased fat accumulation, especially around the stomach area. It also plays a major role in sugar and insulin balance.

**Adrenalin:** This is the acute stress hormone. It increases heart rate, blood pressure, blood sugar and is very potent at breaking down fat to supply fatty acids for energy.

**Estrogen & Progesterone:** These are two female sex hormones present in both men and women that causes cell growth and the production of more cells to enhance fertility. When the body has too much estrogen, it is constantly and unnecessarily multiplying more cells which gives diseases like cancer more opportunity to grow. More important than the body's content of estrogen is its balance with its natural opposing hormone, progesterone. Too much estrogen in a woman will cause her to increase fat storage. If a man is overweight, it is an indication that he is converting more of his testosterone into estrogen.

When estrogen and progesterone are unbalanced and estrogen is dominant, it leads to fat accumulation, weight gain, fluid retention, breast tenderness and cyst formation as well as inflammation in blood vessels contributing to cardiovascular diseases, mood swings, strokes, migraines, carbohydrate cravings, blood sugar problems, insulin imbalances, PMS, prostate cancer, low sperm count and breast or uterine cancer. This imbalance can also depress thyroid and growth hormone function which leads to fatigue and further contributes to excess fat accumulation.

*Hormones Work Synergistically*
These key hormones, along with many other less dominant hormones, all play instrumental roles in managing weight, appetite, mood swings and health. As you can see by their descriptions, each affects the other. Insulin is the most critical because the food you eat has a direct impact on your body's sugar levels which triggers insulin production.

Hormones have major effects on body weight which also influences cholesterol levels. Cholesterol is an essential chemical predominantly made in the liver. Some is also absorbed and manufactured in the intestinal tract. The body maintains good and bad cholesterol which needs to be within safe levels in order to avoid a thickening of the walls of your arteries (arteriosclerosis). When you have your cholesterol checked, the doctor takes a blood test that identifies the amount of good (HDL) and bad (LDL) cholesterol as well as your triglyceride level. Hormones have very powerful effects on cholesterol. Proper cholesterol levels are related to the correct interplay of all your hormones and how harmoniously those hormones are working together. For example, low thyroid, low testosterone and low growth hormone tend to promote elevated cholesterol as does high insulin and high cortisol levels.

If you don't think there is a correlation between hormones and weight management, you are very much mistaken. The number of Americans that are overweight and the percentage of the population that have or are treating hormone-related problems are almost identical. Many of the medications that treat the most common ailments also cause weight gain and fat retention.

**The following is a list of the most commonly treated conditions in America:**

| | | |
|---|---|---|
| **Diabetes:** | 17 million Americans have diabetes | (2000) |
| | 16 million Americans are pre-diabetic | (2000) |
| | 5.9 million unaware they have diabetes | (2000) |
| | 71,252 diabetic deaths each year | (2001) |
| | 23.6 million annual doctor visits for diabetes | (2000) |
| | Average hospital stay of 5.4 days | (1999) |
| **Stroke:** | #3 cause of death | (2000) |
| | 167,661 deaths per year | (2000) |
| | 981,000 inpatient hospital visits per year | (2000) |
| **Prostate:** | 2.8 million cases per year | (2000) |
| | 184,000 prostate removal procedures annually | (2000) |
| | 31,078 prostate deaths per year | (2000) |
| | Accounts for 30% of cancer caused in men | (2003) |
| | Accounts for 11% of deaths in men | (2003) |
| **Thyroid:** | Under-active thyroid #2 most treated ailment | (2002) |
| | Est. 20% of the population goes undiagnosed | (2001) |
| **Hormone Replacement:** | 20 million Americans are on estrogen (HRT) therapy | (2003) |
| | #1 most treated ailment | (2002) |

Six of America's top ten most commonly prescribed drugs address hormone-related problems:

| | | |
|---|---|---|
| #1 | **Premarin** | **Hormone Replacement Therapy** |
| #2 | **Synthroid** | **For under-active thyroid** |
| #3 | **Lipitor** | **For cholesterol** |
| #7 | **Norvasc** | **Channel blocker for heart/stroke prevention** |
| #9 | **Prozac** | **For depression** |
| #10 | **Glucophage** | **For diabetes** |

*The Country Club Diet* addresses the nutritional needs of your hormones and the best foods to supply those needs. Lifestyle and habit also play a role in making the necessary changes needed in order for you to achieve the body you desire. Taking each challenge one-at-a-time, you will soon be armed with all the information required to control your appetite, elevate your metabolism and take charge of your body.

## HOW DID WEIGHT MANAGEMENT GET THIS HARD?

Most people did not gain unwanted pounds and inches overnight. As we get older, our diets change. Babies eat better than toddlers. Toddlers eat better than adolescents. Adolescents eat better than teens. And, as we move through various decades of adulthood, diet and health become more and more a priority. Sometimes we are still fighting many of the bad habits established when we were younger. Those patterns are not easily broken.

Today, weight and fat loss, in some form, is on the minds of most Americans. You cannot go into a supermarket or convenience store and not notice the wide variety of weight loss articles promoted on the front covers of every magazine and sensational newspaper they carry. Yet, the prevalence of obesity in America has increased 61% between 1991 and 2000, *(WIN of National Institute of Diabetes & Digestive & Kidney Diseases, NIDDK 2002\*.)* From 2001 to 2002, it grew by 21% alone! Depending upon their nationality, as many as 65.8% of women and 56.5% of men\* are overweight and diabetes is increasing at a rate of 8% each year. Do you really think our body's nutritional requirements changed so dramatically in the last ten to twenty years? Of course not. But, what did change was our eating habits and the increase in diseases has shown that our bodies are not responding well to that change.

So, what has happened to America? Simple. Time restrictions and advertising. We are bombarded with hundreds of thousands of positive impressions about unhealthy foods every day and encouraged to eat them with great regularity. The grocery store is stocked full of more than 35 THOUSAND items you SHOULD NEVER EAT! Preservatives are a major part of the shelf-life of its products. It enables us to make fewer trips to the store and 'stock up' with minimal fear of waste. As one major chip manufacturer unwittingly disclosed, "Preservatives aid in the shelf life of our products but, unfortunately do not aid in the shelf life of our consumers!"

Chemical additives and hydrogenated fats are killing Americans and altering hormone function. Many of these 'fake fats' are of a molecular composition that our bodies do not recognize, therefore they do not know how to process or even eliminate them. Every kind of preservative and food chemical raises havoc with your hormones. All in the name of convenience, Americans are short-cutting food processing and, as a result, shortcutting the longevity of their life.

Food chemicals and additives are in anything packaged… even things you assume are fresh and healthy like pre-cut lettuce. Pre-cut lettuce is sometimes referred to as 'salad in a bag'. If you have ever purchased this item, which is available in a variety of lettuce options from romaine to exotic endive, you may have noticed how much longer that bag of salad stays 'fresh' in your refrigerator as compared to a plain head of lettuce. Why do you think the fresh lettuce from the head turns brown and goes bad in a matter of days, yet the cut lettuce that was packaged in the bag will stay fresh for weeks? The bag isn't vacuum-packed. We can see the lettuce freely housed inside. The answer? Chemicals. Unhealthy, oftentimes carcinogenic, chemicals. We subject our body to internal toxins and altered hormone function generated by the metabolism of the poor food choices we make every day. Choices that include too much sugar and refined carbohydrates. These foods can be just as poisonous to the body as industrial chemicals.

Back in the early 50's, before fast food, Americans used to unknowingly eat only those chemicals that were associated with the fertilizers used to maintain proper soil conditions. From the 1950's to the 1970's, after our introduction to fast food restaurants, the average American ate three to four pounds of food additives and chemicals per year. Today, some type of chemical additive is used in just about every processed, can, boxed or packaged food we eat. Now, each year, you can expect to consume approximately twenty pounds of chemicals and food additives by dry weight and more than forty pounds if fast, frozen or convenience food is a regular part of your diet!

Most metabolic problems, hormone conditions, diseases, and advanced aging are caused by cumulative free-radical damage fueled by these toxic chemical invaders. Doctors tell us that this toxic load can be attributed to the epidemic of:

◆ Obesity in 65% of the American population
◆ Heart disease, even in young people
◆ Cancers: breast cancer affects one in eight women
◆ Adolescent diabetes
◆ Chronic fatigue
◆ Autism
◆ Attention deficit disorder (ADD)
◆ Crohn's disease

Sugar and its misuse is also a culprit. And, I don't just mean the obvious candies, cakes and cookies. I mean foods that overload the sugar or insulin levels in your body that you think are healthy. Dr. Lewis was also Medical and Nutrition Consultant to the ongoing National Health and Nutritional Examination Survey (NHANES II) conducted by the U.S. government. This important, ongoing study shows how America eats. One of the results showed the foods most consumed in America were:

**#1   white bread, rolls and crackers**
**#2   donuts, cookies and cake**
**#3   alcoholic beverages**

Eleven of the top twenty foods identified as 'America's favorites' are predominantly pure carbohydrates. Carbohydrates make sugar. Sugar increases insulin production. Increased insulin makes you a 'sugar burner' whose body stores fat.

Today, 89% of the calories in a 'Standard American Diet' come from fat and carbohydrates. These statistics can logically be attributed to the food industry's focus on marketing fast and easy carbohydrate food and snack items to the public. This is a formula for disaster and it has occurred with a vengeance. Is it no wonder that, as a result, our population is:

◆ Sicker than ever
◆ Experiencing an epidemic of heart disease, diabetes, asthma, arthritis, cancer, ADD, autism, and auto-immune disease in YOUNG people
◆ Spending almost as much as the military budget on health care

◆     More obese and overweight than ever (66% of Americans)

◆     Living a longer percentage of life afflicted  with more disease

It is scary to think that the average American eats 152 pounds of sugar per year! Now it should make sense why we are seeing an epidemic of diabetes and chronic degenerative diseases that are growing amongst our population at lightening speed. Obesity, which is one area that we can at least attempt to take control, actually has the greatest impact on our poor health. 2 out of 3 Americans are overweight. 1 out of 3 is obese. In 1970, only 1 out of 7 Americans was obese, What are we doing to ourselves?

Good health isn't an accident. It takes work. Sometimes, it takes discipline. Nobody gets bitten by the 'cancer bug' or is hit by the 'diabetes virus'. These are not germs that fly around and infect the unlucky. They are diseases and conditions that we perpetuate by allowing them into our bodies in the form of chemicals and hydrogenated fats or oils oftentimes hidden in our food. These fats and chemicals so negatively affect our bodies that our hormones cannot fight them and get completely out of balance in the attempt. Dr. Lewis and I are not suggesting that eating right will guarantee a long, healthy life. But, we will tell you that it is a much better insurance policy than eating with blinders on, pretending or praying that you won't be 'infected' by illnesses that have already affected family members or friends. We are a product of our environment. Most of us learned bad eating habits as children. It is a well documented fact that overweight children usually have at least one overweight parent. But, bad habits are not genetic. They are learned. And, they can be unlearned. You don't eat your favorite foods. Your favorite foods become the foods you eat. If you have a weight problem, it is most likely not in your genes... it's simply in your jeans.

## SO, WHAT AM I EATING?

According to the Economic Research Service, US Department of Agriculture, the American diet is full of unhealthy overindulgence. In many cases, the rise of high sugar and chemically filled soft drinks, fats, oils, and cheese consumption, is up as much as one and a half times over the same foods eaten in 1970. As of year end 2000, the average American had eaten:

| | |
|---|---|
| 30 | pounds of cheese |
| 15 | pounds of full fat ice cream |
| 7 | pounds of low fat ice cream |
| 10 | pounds of frozen yogurt |
| 135 | pounds of white & whole wheat breads, cereals, pancakes, cakes & cookies |
| 19 | pounds of rice |
| 11 | pounds of pasta |
| 28 | pounds of corn flour, starch & grits |
| 78 | pounds of added fats & oils due to food processing! |
| 35 | pounds of cooking oils |
| 35 | pounds of butter & margarine |
| 152 | pounds of ADDED SUGAR! |
| 111 | pounds of red meat |
| 83 | pounds of poultry & seafood |
| 276 | pounds of fruits & vegetables |
| 16 | gallons of whole & 2% milk |
| 50 | gallons of soda! |
| 10 | gallons of bottled water |
| 27 | gallons of coffee |
| 28 | gallons of beer |
| 9 | gallons of fruit juice |

What a grocery bill! And people say that dieting is expensive! Fat content is so high in the majority of these foods because, as a society, we are eating more highly processed, nutrient depleted 'individual serving' foods than ever before. Frozen dinners, snack items, soups, pasta-in-a-cup and meals-on-the-go type food all come in convenient, 'eat in your car', 'eat on the run' style packaging. We grab food as we can and those foods are generally full of sugars, man-made trans fats and unhealthy additives. Pound-for-pound, they are also more expensive than health food.

We have a crisis here! The morbidity and mortality of Americans attributable to their overweight condition is approaching that of cigarettes and we're blaming outside influences instead of taking personal responsibility for what we eat. The crime is that most unhealthy medical conditions are preventable by proper lifestyle and dietary choices. Eating too much sugar, either in dessert and snack form or in the form of starchy carbohydrates can cause:

◆ Overweight and obesity
◆ Hormonal infertility and menstrual problems
◆ Diabetes
◆ GI tract dysfunction: Leaky Gut Syndrome leading to a host of diseases such as allergy, asthma, and autoimmune diseases
◆ Immune dysfunction: cancer, thyroiditis
◆ Insulin Resistance: Syndrome X - high bad cholesterol, obesity, high blood pressure, heart disease
◆ Bad Eicosonoids: Arachidonic acid/inflammation/arthritis/blood clots, heart attacks
◆ Glycosolation of proteins: Sugar directly damages the body's proteins and enzymes leading to skin wrinkling, cataracts, and premature aging
◆ Blockage of vitamin C absorption
◆ Candida - causing cravings, sharp mood and energy swings
◆ Feeds cancer cells: Cancer cells can only live on sugar!
◆ Increases the production of adrenaline which leads to increased cholesterol and all the harmful effects of chronic stress

As a society, we cannot assume that because an item looks healthy, it is. Or, that because it is a 'coffee drink' it must be OK. People are unwittingly eating 600-calorie 'health muffins', 700 calorie tuna sandwiches and 800 calorie café-Frappuccinos without thought to what they are doing to their body. If all they ate were these three items in one day, they would have consumed 2100 empty calories and still felt like they ate practically nothing. If they added dinner to the mix, they would have eaten well over 3500 calories in a single day but would still wonder why they "can't lose any weight." It isn't the calorie count that becomes the issue in this example, it is the empty quality of the calories that we are addressing.

We already know that sugar isn't good for us. But, did you stop to think about the fact that it is actually killing you in the process of compromising health and productivity? Sugar is simply empty calories which means they lack the nutrients, minerals and vitamins required for their own metabolism. They deplete the body's storage of nutrients and interfere with its energy production, fat metabolism, heat production, and activity. The results you may see are a decreased metabolism, slow fat burning, fatigue, obesity, cancer, diabetes and premature aging.

Pay attention! What you eat affects the way your body functions. Would you continue to put spoons down your garbage disposal when you know they burn up the blades, making the effective performance of the disposal almost impossible? Doesn't your body deserve the same consideration?

I think, sometimes, in our fear of all the potential diseases that face us, we think we can avoid these conditions by pretending they don't exist. Why should someone's report of a high cholesterol level come as much of a shock when they live on breakfast bagels, hoagies and pasta? What did they THINK would result? Wasn't the fact that their pants didn't fit anymore provide the clue that all was not well?

I'm not trying to make you defensive. The fact is, weight is merely a symptom of a much greater problem. We have worked with hundreds of thousands of people who avoid snacks and try to 'eat right' but have fallen victim to the misinformation and food hype that sells products. As a nation, we are not intentionally malnourished and overweight. We are much smarter than that. We are simply lacking the information that the business of 'Big Food' does not want us to know. That changes right now.

## THE DANGERS OF AMERICA'S 10 MOST POPULAR FOODS

No one argues that today's fast-paced environment makes proper eating difficult. It is a lot easier to make good food choices when you begin to understand the ramifications of poor ones. People are under the misconception that we eat our favorite foods. The fact is, the foods we eat BECOME our favorites because that is what we become accustomed to. We can all change our taste buds and our attitude toward unhealthy food when armed with the right information.

Anyone who once drank whole milk is well aware of their first reaction to 2% or skim. The 'new' milk looked gray, watery and very unappealing. But, anyone who made the transition to the lighter milk now finds whole milk too heavy. Taste buds can change. We are all victims of habit. Generally, we tend to eat the same basic food most of the time.  For many, the idea of eliminating what they consider to be a food staple seems almost impossible.  That is, however, until they learn what some of their 'daily favorites' are doing to their body and to their health.

What you decide to eat is certainly your business.   But, at least do it 'heads-up'. Don't pretend you are not poisoning yourself when you choose to eat things that are clearly unhealthy.  Cancer, diabetes and heart disease don't just happen.  YOU 'grow them' in your body by feeding and encouraging their growth and development with carcinogenic chemicals and unnatural sugar consumption oftentimes hidden in your 'favorite foods'.

The following is a listing of the top ten most popular foods eaten in America.  We have disclosed information about each one that will most likely surprise you and may even affect how you order the next time you find yourself in a fast-food restaurant.

### 1, 2 & 3. Hamburgers, Hot Dogs & Chicken Nuggets (6):

- All considered "high risk" foods because of the poor health standards under which they are manufactured.
- The time consuming process for making processed meats creates high bacteria counts and putrefaction of the meat which need to be treated with chemicals.
- Putrefaction causes meat to turn green which is then dyed with red chemicals to appear fresh.  Unless marked otherwise, hamburger will always contain red dyes.
- Hamburgers, hotdogs and chicken nuggets are made with the unusable, worst leftovers of the slaughterhouse… much of which comes right off the floor.  Any meat 'part' that cannot be sold on its own merit is ground up and used for burger.  This includes hooves, bone, snout, ears and other animal parts.
- Because burger parts all come from the animal, "pure beef" can be used on the label.  The same holds true for chicken nuggets - even if feet & beak are part of the ingredients!
- Most of America's top 3 favorites contain the flavor enhancer, "MSG" (monosodium glutamate) which causes headaches and allergic reactions.  MSG is a chemical used to fatten up laboratory animals and will ultimately make you fat when consumed.
- The beef industry is the largest user of antibiotics in the world.

◆ Antibiotics offser the dangerous bacteria housed in its animals. This has resulted in a widespread occurrence of infection-resistance to antibiotics.

◆ Ground beef is more likely to harbor life-threatening E-coli than any other food.

◆ Hamburgers are the single biggest food item that inflicts the most damage on the American diet.... billions served.... billions spent on doctor visits and hospital bills.

◆ The hormones fed to cattle and chickens can make you fat through the consumption of their meat and cause an imbalance in your hormonal make-up.

◆ A Cheeseburger contains more than 100% of your TOTAL daily recommended fat intake!

◆ Burger King's Double Whopper with Cheese has 1150 calories and 76 grams of fat with 33 of them saturated, plus a whopping 1,530 mg. of sodium!

◆ Burger condiments like pickle, lettuce and tomato are treated with cancer-causing chemical sulfites that are used to maintain a false freshness in the vegetables.

◆ Most burgers contain 1090 mg of sodium, (45% of daily recommended Daily Value), and can promote water retention.

◆ Hot dogs have nitrites which are thought to cause stomach cancer, and leukemia. Fillers and non-meat binders used to hold hot dog meat together can be anything from cereal, non-fat dry milk, or soy which adds more carbohydrates and processed ingredients.

◆ Synthetic collagen casings are used to form and shape hot dogs.

◆ Hot dogs contain up to 40% of its content in undisclosed saturated fats.

◆ When the buns are baked, they release a powerful toxin called acrylimides which is a known carcinogen that causes nerve damage.

◆ Nuggets & Tenders are usually made from unusable chicken parts and rarely made from whole white meat although it is bleached to look like it is.

◆ A typical 340 calorie serving of Nuggets or Tenders is typically 50% fat.

◆ Nuggets & Tenders are heavily breaded for substance. Very high carbohydrate content.

◆ Some chicken nuggets contain aluminum which is toxic to the brain and poisons the metabolism.

◆ Nuggets & Tenders are deep fried in oxidized oil that is re-used for weeks at a time!

### 4. French Fries:
◆ French fries are very toxic.
◆ In order to make French fries, they must be cooked at high temperatures which causes the chemical, acrylimide to be released.
◆ Potatoes are grown in the ground and have a higher pesticide absorption level than almost any other food product.
◆ Fries are cooked in oxidized oil that is re-used for weeks at a time.
◆ Potatoes have a very high glycemic index meaning it turns to sugar very quickly in the body. Eating a baked potato (or equivalent quantity of French fries) has the same sugar equivalent as a large piece of chocolate cake!
◆ Full of undisclosed trans fats.

### 5. Oreo Cookies: *THE NUMBER ONE COOKIE IN AMERICA (6 cookies = serving size)*
◆ Predominantly made up of 23 grams of straight-line sugar.
◆ Chocolate is LAST ingredient listed which means chocolate is the least of the ingredients.
◆ 370 empty calories with almost no nutritional benefits - you could eat 2 whole chicken breasts for the same amount of calories!
◆ 6 cookies have 12 grams of fat, 2.5 grams of saturated fat and 40 carbs - more than 50% of your daily carbohydrate allowance in only 6 cookies.
◆ Oreo cookies will set you up for craving more sugar within 2-3 hours.
◆ 'Natural flavors' are manufactured chemicals to make Oreos taste like great chocolate cookies. Highly processed foods have these flavor enhancers which are nothing more than carcinogenic chemicals with no natural flavors of their own.
◆ The Nabisco Company refused to disclose how many trans fats there are in Oreo cookies - they termed that information as "classified"!
◆ High sugar content. Sugar causes facial wrinkles and dimples the skin.

### 6. Pizza:
◆ Commercial pizzas are made exclusively of 5 genetically modified foods:
  • *Cheese 'food' (Contains only 10% cheese - it cannot even be called real cheese)*
  • *Enriched white flour which has been bleached of natural vitamins and minerals BUT has been 'enriched' by adding back a miniscule amount of synthetic vitamins.*

- *Tomato sauce made from tomato-like substances that produce their own pesticides, IN YOU.*
- *Wheat in the pizza crust is genetically modified.*
- *Contains cottonseed oil. Cotton is not a "food", therefore it can be sprayed with any chemical or pesticide farmers choose. The seed carries most of the poison of the cotton plant. The USDA and the FDA do not cooperate with each other in making sure this oil is safe to eat. It is not. Plus, it is highly hydrogenated and dangerous to your health.*

◆ Pizza is baked at such a high temperature, the crust will form cancer-causing acrylimides.

◆ Pepperoni & sausage toppings are 'high risk,' processed meats which add lots of nitrites, chemicals, preservatives, and saturated fats.

## 7. Soda:

◆ The active ingredient in Coke is phosphoric acid. On the Ph scale, it is very acidic and can dissolve a nail in about 4 days.

◆ High acid content in the body makes it very difficult to lose weight.

◆ Soda will leach the calcium out of bones and promotes osteoporosis.

◆ There are 10-12 teaspoons of empty calorie sugar in one can of soda.

◆ Diet sodas with artificial sweeteners will promote sugar cravings because sweeteners are 'sweeter' than sugar.

◆ Colorings used in sodas are cancer-causing.

◆ Soda is called 'liquid candy' because of its high sugar content. It is the equivalent of drinking a candy bar!

◆ High fructose corn syrup, a major ingredient:
- *Damages proteins.*
- *Is stored in the body as fat.*
- *Is made from corn, which is a modified food that produces its own pesticides.*

## 8. Ice Cream:

◆ High in fat content. 1 serving (usually 4 ounces!) can provide as much as 50% of your recommended fat for the day.

◆ High in carbohydrates. 1 serving provides almost 40% of your total recommended carbohydrate intake for the day.

◆ High in sugar which promotes sugar cravings and causes skin to wrinkle and dimple.

◆ Full of hydrogenated and trans fats which are unnatural and causes:
  - *elevate cholesterol*
  - *clog arteries*
  - *create free radicals (which may cause cancer)*

◆ Hormones put into cows to increase milk production will slow your metabolism and can cause breast and ovarian tumors, cysts and cancer.

## 9. Donuts:

◆ The average donut contains approximately 300 calories.

◆ 1 donut provides more than 50% of your recommended daily carbohydrate intake.

◆ High in salt content which will promote water retention.

◆ Donuts are deep fried in oxidized oil that is re-used for weeks at a time.
  - *Dunkin Donuts changes the oil every 300 dozen!*
  - *Oils at high temperatures develop rancidity and free radicals which can:*
  - Poison and slow metabolism
  - Seriously threaten health.
  - High sugar content promotes sugar cravings and ages skin.

## 10. Potato Chips: America's #1 Snack Food

Today, Americans consume more potato chips than any other people in the world. As a world food, potatoes are second in human consumption only to rice.

◆ It takes 4 pounds of potatoes to make 1 pound of potato chips.

◆ Very calorie dense. A small 2 oz. bag has over 300 calories.

◆ Potato chips are deep fried in oxidized oil that is re-used for weeks at a time!

◆ Deep fried at high temperatures which cause the chemical, acrylimide to be released.
  - *When you eat 1 single serving bag of potato chips you may be eating up to 500 times more acrylamide than the maximum level allowed in drinking water.*
  - *A single potato chip could contain as much acrylamide as is allowed for an 8-ounce glass of drinking water!*
  - *High in hidden saturated fats.*
  - *High sodium/salt content promotes water retention.*

## "HEALTHY CHIPS" LIKE BAKED LAYS OR THOSE CONTAINING OLESTRA CAN BE MORE DANGEROUS TO YOUR HEALTH THAN REGULAR CHIPS.

◆ Baked Lays, almost as calorie dense as original Lays, are a highly processed mixture of dehydrated potato and food starch pressed into a chip shape, full of carcinogenic chemicals.

◆ Olean/Olestra potato chips., can cause 'anal oil leakage' or a variety of gastrointestinal problems, as reported on the bag.

◆ Block fat absorption which alters your body's ability to absorb valuable nutrients contained in the healthy foods you eat.

  • *Stops the body from properly absorbing carotenoids and other valuable phytochemicals that protect your body from heart disease, cancer and macular degeneration.*

"How does the government let this happen?" you might ask. Simple. Food is big business. Trans fats, which are dangerous manufactured fats used to increase the shelf-life of products, are not even listed on nutritional food labels. In fact, it will not be until sometime in the future that the government will require the disclosure of trans fats to the public. At this time, big food companies are fighting this act because they do not want the consumer's attention to be drawn to a negative footnote that may affect sales. According to a December 2002 article in *The Wall Street Journal,* a lobbyist for Grocer Manufacturers of America was quoted as saying, "The food label is a place for quantitative information. Its purpose is not to provide nutritional counseling." In other words, 'let's tell the public as little as possible'.

In your quest for good health, question anything that does not appear to be logical. Does it really make sense that a cookie or Twinkie can stay "fresh" for over a year as long as it remains packaged? How can that be? Home-made cakes and cookies can't stay fresh for more than about a week. Why then is it possible that manufactured cookies & cakes are so magical that they can stay fresh for months and months?

As a nation we are in denial of the obvious fact that manufacturers use chemical intervention to increase their product's shelf-life and it saves them money. It has appeared for years that we'd rather eat the cookie or cupcake in blind bliss. But, would we? Everyone wants to live a long healthy life. Help your body make your life-expectancy goal a reality instead of working against it. Good eating is a matter of choice... Make the right one!

# WEIGHT LOSS IS NOT A BEHAVIOR, IT'S AN OUTCOME

Successful weight loss is a result of appropriate behaviors and eating habits that allow your body to function efficiently. It is one of many positive outcomes that you will experience during this program. It is critical that you recognize all of the many successful effects that are a direct result of your fat loss efforts. When you are aware of the totality of your success, you will be much more encouraged. Look for:

| | | | |
|---|---|---|---|
| 📄 | More energy | * | Increased self-esteem |
| 📄 | Better health | * | Improved medical reports |
| 📄 | Fewer cravings | * | More confidence |
| 📄 | Less fear of food | * | Better sleep |
| 📄 | Clothes fit better | * | Fewer aches & pains |
| 📄 | Feel sexier | * | Enjoy exercise |

Mental preparation is essential for your ability to self-change. When you recognize the value of certain behaviors throughout this process, you can mentally establish those behaviors as your own. You can use the following list to encourage your progress and solidify your commitment to change:

- Your body needs to be nutritionally balanced in order to function and be healthy.
- Your weight problem is not your fault.
- Food alone is deficient in many of the nutrients the body needs.
- Exercise needs to be a part of a healthy lifestyle.
- Diets don't work. New eating patterns need to be developed that are satisfying, fit into lifestyle requirements and are healthy.
- Focus meals on proteins, fruits & vegetables. Minimize starches & dairy.
- You can learn to prefer to eat healthier food.
- Cravings can be avoided.
- 64 ounces of water must be consumed daily.
- Food is not to be used as a reward or as a solution to problems.
- You can achieve anything you set your mind to.

**SELF-EVALUATION.** Self-changers must be aware of all facets of their health, emotions and behaviors. This may be the first time that you have openly assessed how you feel both physically and emotionally in many different situations. To help identify problem triggers, you need to recall your actions and emotions just prior to any negative behaviors. Understanding oneself; how you act, feel, relate, and handle negative, stressful or even celebration situations is critical to changing behaviors that conflict with your desired outcome.

Be aware, your overweight condition has served its purpose in your life so you can now let go of it and all of the behaviors that keep it with you. You possess the personal power and free will needed to take control over your own life. When it comes to self-changing, you can do whatever you decide and are willing to do. Asking "why me?" won't change your weight or your health, but asking "what can I do?" will. That is the first step.

Change requires the elimination of certain thought patterns that may have kept you stuck in your current condition:

- I'm a victim of…
- I'm entitled to…
- Someone else needs to repair this…
- Who can I blame this on?…

Unhappiness with your appearance, no matter how subtle your awareness, can be very self-defeating. If you have gone on numerous diets or have regained unwanted pounds and inches over the years, it is natural for you to fear failure when starting yet another plan. Or, your fear may be over more than just the possibility of an unsuccessful diet. It may go much deeper. The good news is that you can use your fears as a motivator to make you take action. Let your fear now become the overwhelming culmination of all the potential results that remaining in an overweight state may create such as:

- loss of self-esteem
- lack of personal control
- becoming undesirable to your mate
- loss of sensuality
- complex health issues
- hopelessness
- high medical expenses

You can't wage war against your weight problems. The best way to overcome any circumstance you view as undesirable is to attack it positively. When you tell yourself that you hate how you look, hate what you eat, hate exercise and hate diets, you surround yourself with negative energy that literally retards your problem-solving ability. Failure only occurs when you quit trying. Even Thomas Edison felt he never experienced failure during his first thousand attempts to invent the light bulb. By his own accounts, 'he simply identified a thousand ways that did not work!' If you think about it, you have not failed at your previous attempts to lose weight either. Your success simply wasn't as big a priority in your life then as it is now.

Being stressed, anxious or depressed over your health and appearance will not help you reach your goal. According to three separate studies featured in the British Journal of Medical Psychology (1988 Vol 61) "Stress is more closely related to heart disease and to cancer, than smoking." These studies prove that if you can 'think yourself sick' you can also 'think yourself well' too. Researchers learned that when people experience positive emotions, it increased their problem-solving ability and mental focus which released more of their brain's primary "feel good" hormone, dopamine. Good thoughts trigger the body's ability to feel good in return.

Building health is the optimum way to defeat illness and accomplish your goals. 60,000 American die each year from illegal drugs, but at least 250,000 die from overeating and being sedentary. You posses the ability, (even though you may not know it) to change the way you look and feel. You just need to be ready.

If you've ever known anyone who quit smoking cold-turkey, and never had the desire to start smoking again, you were viewing someone who focused their attention on the positive results associated with being an ex-smoker rather than lamenting and missing the fact that they were attempting to remove cigarettes from their life. If you want to change the way you eat and improve your health, then you must constantly focus on the benefits of that wise choice rather than on the inner conflict you may experience when you consider change. It is all a matter of perspective. You won't miss behaviors that have not served you well in the past unless you choose to miss them.

## ATTITUDE IS EVERYTHING

Mentally prepare yourself. During each weakening or self-defeating time that pops up during your weight loss period, take a few minutes (like 3-5) to mentally remind yourself of all the positive qualities you possess:

- you're a loving person...
- you consider others...
- you're organized...
- you keep a nice house...
- you're honest and dependable...
- you're a great parent...
- you're fun...
- you have family and friends who love you....
- life is important to you.

Make your personal list of attributes as long as possible. You might even want to write your list down as a reminder and keep it in your wallet so you can refer to it when you get upset with yourself or turn to food as a comfort mechanism. Surely you can see as you look down your list that a person as wonderful as yourself deserves to look and feel the way your heart desires.

Whatever caused you to gain weight in the first place is yesterday's news. Today is a new day. Being overweight is nothing to feel guilty about. There are a zillion reasons why you are heavier than you would like to be. Aging alone can be the cause of as much as a ten pound gain each year and you certainly can't stop time from moving forward. Even if food was used as a coping mechanism during a very difficult period in your life, be appreciative that food got you through the challenging time, but over-indulging is no longer needed anymore. Recognize that food can now become your sustenance, not your solace.

If you have used your overweight as an excuse over the years, now is the time to acknowledge that fact and move on. Some people have told me they hid behind their overweight condition and used it:

- to not participate in some activities
- as an excuse to not exercise
- to show a visible confirmation of their self-perceived flaws
- to punish themselves or their partner

Once you identify the power you once gave to your condition and remove it, it no longer has power over your ability to change it.

For most people, overweight creates a certain anxiety. It is hard to be truly happy when you're unhappy with your appearance or concerned about your health. Even identifying and appreciating all of the benefits your overweight condition created

Shelbyville-Shelby County Public Library

at one time or another will help you recognize that you no longer need to fear shedding unwanted pounds. Your excess weight no longer has a purpose, so be grateful that you made it through the experience unscathed. Assuming you subscribe to the theory, 'There is a lesson in every circumstance we experience in our lifetime...' your overweight condition may have taught you a lot over the years such as:

- food awareness
- it helped to educate you about nutrition and reading labels
- you now know your problems cannot be resolved by overindulging with food
- eating right isn't really that hard
- you have options and can lose weight if you really want to
- your family and friends have always loved you unconditionally

If you have decided to take charge of your body, focus your thinking on what you want, not what you don't want...on what you should eat, not what you shouldn't. When you think about how you want to look and feel, you will begin to act and eat in a manner that reinforces what you want - a new body! When you think like a healthy, fit individual, your desire to eat like a depressed, overweight one will rapidly dissolve. Before you know it, you will become the physical person in health and appearance that you first created in your mind. It really is that simple.

Knowledge is power. The more you know how food works and what is good for you, the easier it will be for you to make better choices when it comes to food selection. It is equally important for you to understand how your body operates so you are better able to identify signs that might indicate imbalances or less than optimal body function. The more you know, the easier it will be to break bad habits that have kept you trapped in a body you no longer enjoy. It is now up to you.

**FAMILY EVALUATION.** Close friends or family members can be a positive and helpful part of your 'team of helpers'. During this process you may want to ask some of them to evaluate or provide insights to your eating and lifestyle patterns. Your 'helper' will assist your getting a more complete picture of yourself and help to identify any problem in areas of which you may be unaware. Seeing yourself through another person's eyes can be very enlightening.

**CONSIDER NUTRITIONAL SUPPLEMENTS.** It is almost impossible to achieve complete and balanced nutrition from traditional food sources alone. Proper nutrition is an important element for hormone balance and fat loss, but simply cutting calories or eating 'right' is not enough to achieve the body you desire. Research shows that little of the fruits and vegetables grown today have any nutritional resemblance to those grown 50 years ago. Unfortunately, the fruits and vegetables we eat now have been grown in depleted soil void of magnesium, selenium, chromium, other important nutrients and therefore, have very poor nutritional value. Even protein sources like beef, chicken and fish can be full of artificial hormones, chemicals or toxic metals like mercury. In fact, most grown foods are often 80-90% depleted of the critical minerals and vitamins our bodies need in order to metabolize food and process it efficiently enough to maintain healthy weight. Americans are perpetually in a nutritionally depleted state which makes weight loss and good health almost impossible.

Food, in the form of multivitamins, antioxidants, greens, protein powders and the like should be a part of your physical fortification and nutritional balancing plan. These are neither medications nor drugs. They are natural sources of food in concentrated forms that should be taken regularly with meals. You should be sure to check with your personal physician to confirm that the supplements you select are safe in combination with any prescribed medications you may be taking. It is critical that you understand that it may be necessary for you to take a variety of supplements that, in no way, indicates you are ill or being medicated. Pills, capsules & powders are merely an efficient delivery system that provides appropriate dosages of daily required nutrients without the associated calories or inefficiencies of food items. They do not replace eating real food. They simply boost the body's nutrition for optimum hormone balance and good health.

**SUCCESS AWARENESS.** Along the way, I want you to concentrate on duplicating those behaviors that you know help create your desired outcome. During this course, you will be asked to identify behaviors that have historically been counterproductive in achieving the desired health and weight goal you seek. Once identified, there will be no need to repeat those behaviors because the predictable result will surely follow. By maintaining a success awareness, you will be less likely to feel defeated or to relapse into historical patterns once again.

Everyone experiences good and bad food days. Minimizing bad eating habits and maximizing good ones is your goal. A bad food day does not indicate a failure of the program or your personal efforts. Guilt, remorse, shame, and embarrassment can all trigger anxiety and depression that can lead to self-sabotage and defeat.

Being aware of this potential will help you overcome it before it happens and you can continue to move forward.

I cannot stress enough that, in order to be effective and maintainable, behavior and dietary changes need to be made gradually. Developing your personal plan for needed change and easing into the various requirements of that plan will enable you to feel both empowered and successful. Regardless of your enthusiasm, you should not make too many changes until you are mentally and physically prepared to do so. You didn't gain weight overnight. Do not expect to lose it unrealistically fast.

The key element of success for this or any weight loss program is establishing the confidence that the plan you have embarked upon is both sensible and workable. Fads or diets promising rapid results may work temporarily but, unless the underlying behaviors that caused your weight gain are addressed, the excess weight lost by unrealistic, short-term calorie reduction diets can and will eventually return. Once confidence in a realistic and practical program is established, the only thing left for you to do is to believe in your ability to succeed. Then, make a commitment to accept nothing less than success. There are no 'quick fix' solutions to weight management. A complicated set of parental influences during adolescence, health and food misinformation, personal responsibilities and lifestyle issues have all conspired to add undesired pounds on your body over the years. It will take time to identify these factors, neutralize them and reconstruct positive behaviors that will become part of an automatic response system resulting in permanent life-long weight control.

It is critical that you and your 'team of helpers' be patient and maintain a positive, 'can do' attitude throughout this process. You need to address the reason behind any block you may feel toward your plan. For example, if lowering carbohydrates is proving too difficult for you, then you need to reevaluate and increase your carbohydrates to a more maintainable level until you are better prepared to lower them to the level they need to be. In this way you will recognize that the program is flexible and that you have done nothing 'wrong' by not following your personal directives exactly. Additionally, if you feel that you are doing everything correctly and weight loss is not as evident as it should be, it is time to seek additional assistance from your doctor. Perhaps you have a food sensitivity or serious physical imbalance that is blocking your ability to lose weight. The body is a complicated, chemically driven machine that can falter for any number of reasons. Our objective is to address the common, easily correctible deficiencies and imbalances you are experiencing that led you to purchase this book.

# HOW THE BODY WORKS

When the body is overweight or in poor health, it affects every organ, every hormone, every joint and every system throughout the anatomy. In order to control weight, all body functions must be working harmoniously. Simply addressing the need for appetite control, for example, will not provide the body with the balance it needs to properly manage its weight. Appetite is simply one of many factores. To best explain the synergistic relationship all parts have with one another, I am going to use a broken toe as an example:

When someone breaks their toe, it affects the way they walk. Adjusting where they put their weight can affect their ankle, knees, hips, back and even the opposite leg. Pain, in non-related areas like the back, can be directly attributed to the single broken toe.

When it comes to fat loss, your body is no different. If your metabolic system is not active, if sugar levels run too high, if your body is full of toxins or malnourished, weight loss is almost impossible. Yet, traditionally, we relate weight loss only with what we put into our mouths.

### Did You Know That Stress CAN CAUSE Obesity Too?
Stress is a major factor contributing to obesity and most likely plays a significant role in the lives of most of us. If you describe yourself as a 'stress eater', you most likely assume that eating as a comfort mechanism when you are stressed is how stress can cause an overweight condition. The truth is, stress WITHOUT overindulgence or "stress eating" will still slow the metabolism and cause weight gain all by itself. It is more obvious to most people how stress contributes to heart disease, diabetes, asthma, ulcers, and other maladies. However, stress actually re-shapes and re-contours your body by increasing fat accumulation while decreasing muscle mass which leads to a saggy and bumpy physique. This stress-induced reshaping will appear as increased fat, especially around hips, thighs and tummy with a simultaneous loss of muscle.

It is important that you do not confuse the relationship between stress and overeating. Overeating is obvious with obvious results and is regularly a comfort mechanism for stress. But, this physical stress-connection is much more subtle. You don't have to be a 'stress eater' for your body to adversely respond to stress.

Modern life is full of stress. We see this at all ages, but it is especially intense from age 30 through 50 when there is stress derived from one's job, financial concerns, children, family, parents, college, school, or even everyday stresses that encompass everything from rude co-workers to getting cut off in traffic. Even though some stressors appear to last for mere minutes, to dissipate their profound effects can take up to two weeks! In that period, numerous other problems further accelerate stress levels. These issues can physically re-shape your body and make you fat. As a defense mechanism, body fat goes up even though you have not changed eating habits or activity levels.

**Chronic stress can have the following hormonal effects:**

- ◆ Increased cortisol which causes fat accumulation in stomach, hips and promotes loss of muscle mass
- ◆ Decreased thyroid function which leads to slow metabolism and slow fat burn thus increasing fat accumulation
- ◆ Increased insulin resistance and insulin level. (Insulin is the fat storage hormone so we do not burn fat, but rather store it.)
- ◆ Decreased growth hormone which causes decreased fat breakdown and decreased muscle mass (sarcopenia).
- ◆ Decreased muscle mass causes decreased fat burning because muscle is the major fat burner. (Muscle is the major fat burner because it is loaded with mitochondria which are the energy factories of the body.)
- ◆ Decreased muscle leads to decreased activity, decreased exercise, decreased energy use, and increased fatigue.
- ◆ Increased cholesterol, triglycerides and blood pressure, causes fatigue and sleep problems.

The result of chronic stress mirrors the aging process. Stress, all by itself, ages you. When this negative influence is controlled, you can live a longer, healthier and thinner life. But, stress must be controlled. You cannot change the external stressors, however, how you handle and react to them determines your hormonal response and overall health. Reaction to stress does not have to be negative and stress does not solve any problems. Challenges are simply tasks that must be handled. You must learn to keep stress in perspective while learning how to control the harmful effects of stressors so you are better able to take control of your own life.

# INSULIN - THE MASTER HORMONE

Back in the 1500's and 1600's, when sugar was rare, the wealthy used to have clandestine 'sugar parties' to get 'high'. They knew that sugar blackened their teeth, but what it did to the inside of their body, no one was able to see. Your body performs with zero sugar intake because the body can make all the sugar it needs from fats, proteins, and complex carbohydrates. Let me give you an example of the affects of sugar that I think most of us relate to:

Anyone who has children or whoever babysat a child who had a cookie or ice cream for dessert prior to their arrival, will fully understand the influence sugar has on the body. In this example I am going to demonstrate the impact sugar consumption can have on an 8 year old child. The average 8 year old with a normal blood sugar level has about 5 grams of sugar in their entire bloodstream. That is what a healthy 8 year old system should have. If that child drinks 1 soda, however, they have now added as much as 40 grams of sugar to their blood system - 6-8 times more than what naturally exists. If you consider the average child has a sugar frosted cereal for breakfast, a soda for lunch, candy bar in the afternoon and a soda plus dessert at dinner, they will have consumed, in one day, the blood sugar necessary to sustain 20 or more children!

It is no wonder that behavior problems, attention deficits, lack of focus, poor memory retention and juvenile diabetes is at an all time high among our children. Dr. Oscar Rasmussen conducted a study with school children not long ago. He gave them a specific exam in the morning and a similar exam in the afternoon. The afternoon exam came shortly after the children had eaten a Twinkie and soda for lunch. The reported decline in the performance and accuracy of the tested children after having eaten the Twinkie & soda was 16-20% LOWER than it had been when the children were tested without sugar foods that same morning.

The adult body is no different. Its response to sugar is just as dramatic as the example given for the 8 year old child. The amount of sugar needed to sustain an adult body is not much more than that of the 8 year old. At the beginning of the Twentieth Century, Americans consumed between five and ten pounds of sugar each year. Today we are consuming 150-175 pounds annually!

## Insulin Affects Everything And It's Not About Diabetes
Most of us assume that insulin is something that only affects diabetics. We don't relate to it as having anything to do with a 'healthy' person. But, that's not true.

Insulin is the master hormone in your body. It is so powerful that the body has five hormones: glucagon, growth hormone, adrenaline, noradrenaline, and cortisone, just to counter-balance its effects. Insulin is responsible for managing how your body uses the sugars and starches from the food you eat. It is the 'storage hormone'. When insulin balance is disrupted, starches and sugars are turned into fat rather than being burned as a fuel. Both sweets, like desserts and candy, as well as starches like potato or bread affect insulin levels in the body.

- Insulin is the major cause of most weight problems and fat loss dilemmas.
- An insulin imbalance will cause your body to store and retain fat.
- Insulin imbalance causes increased appetite.
- Insulin is created by eating sugars OR starches - both sources can be equally damaging
- You do NOT need to eat sweets in order to have insulin problems.

When insulin balance in the body becomes disrupted, the starches and sugars you eat turn into fat.

- Elevated insulin converts sugar & starch into fat instead of burning fat as fuel.
- Elevated insulin prevents utilization and breakdown of fat causing it to be stored.
- Elevated insulin inhibits other hormones that are normally used to break down fat and increase metabolism.
- Elevated insulin can slow the metabolism by indirectly decreasing thyroid activity.
- Elevated insulin accelerates aging and chronic degenerative diseases.

High levels of insulin, sometimes referred to as the 'death hormone,' are very damaging to the body and contribute to:

- strokes
- heart attacks
- diabetes
- cancer
- arthritis
- numerous inflammatory diseases

When you have a history of weight loss difficulty and you answer "Yes" to any of the following questions, you have a problem. You are potentially taking a very dangerous sugar-insulin-adrenalin-serotonin roller coaster ride.

- Do you eat when nervous, depressed or bored, rather than hungry?
- Are you intensely hungry between meals?
- Are you irritable or feel shaky when hungry?
- Does your fatigue disappear after eating?
- Do you feel faint or have heart palpitations if meals are delayed?
- Do you have strong cravings for sweets like chocolate or desserts?
- Does your energy level and mood fluctuate drastically?
- Do you lie about how much sweet food you eat?
- Is a headache or crankiness suddenly relieved by something sweet?
- Do you carry candy with you 'just in case'?
- Do you have trouble with concentration or memory?

Your goal should be to keep insulin levels as stable as possible by eating balanced meals throughout the day. Breakfast, lunch and dinner are all important meals while regulating the amount of high-insulin-producing foods you eat. Most people will need to convert from a carbohydrate-based diet to a protein based one in order to get their insulin levels balanced. That is what The Country Club Diet is all about.

### *How Does Insulin Work In A Balanced Body?*

As we have discussed, food is made up of carbohydrates, proteins and fats. All three affect your blood sugar, but carbohydrates have the most dramatic effect. Carbohydrates are broken down and absorbed into your bloodstream in the form of sugar or glucose, raising your blood sugar level. When this occurs, the pancreas secretes insulin to transport the sugar in your blood into your body's cells where it is burned as fuel for energy production. If there is too much sugar or insulin, the excess is stored as fat. Insulin acts like a "chemical key" that opens up cell membranes allowing sugar or glucose to enter. This process naturally lowers the amount of sugar left circulating in the blood. In a healthy individual, glucose and insulin rise and fall gradually in the blood, both in sync with each other. When the levels of sugar become low, you feel hungry and eat more. Then, the cycle begins all over again.

### What Happens When Insulin Is Out Of Balance?

Overages of glucose or sugar that are not burned as fuel, stored in the liver or stored in muscle tissue for future use, is converted to fat. This mechanism is thrown out of balance for a variety of reasons:

- ❖ High insulin
- ❖ Excess carb or sugar intake
- ❖ Conditions of overweight
- ❖ Thyroid imbalances
- ❖ Diabetes

Any one of these reasons can cause most of the glucose or sugar in your blood to be converted into fat. When this occurs, changes in glucose and insulin levels are much more sudden and extreme. Insulin spikes tend to temporarily raise serotonin, the "feel good" hormone. As levels drop, people feel let down and then crave carbohydrates to raise serotonin again. Even though the excess insulin creates an imbalance, the body now wants more. When you eat more starches or sugars to satisfy your cravings, the body responds by surging insulin into the bloodstream in order to transport the sugar to where it can be stored as fat. When the sugar has been transported out of the bloodstream and into the fat storage areas which are typically hips, thighs, stomach and buttocks, the sugar "high" is gone and your mood level crashes again.

### Sugar Cravings Identify An Imbalance

The body's rapid rise in insulin not only brings about a sugar crash, it keeps blood sugar levels low by preventing or blocking the conversion of fat back into sugar or glucose. Your body is burning sugar and, by doing so, is creating a hormonal change and tendency toward a low blood sugar level, called "hypoglycemia." Low blood sugar will leave you feeling fatigued, light-headed, irritable, nervous and depressed. In order to feel good again, the cycle must start all over. As the sugar goes down, your body puts out adrenaline, glucagon, and other hormones, which then cause you to be nervous, shaky, cold, sweaty, have palpitations or tremors. Sound familiar?

This insulin rise and fall constitutes what some in the medical community refer to as the sugar-insulin-adrenaline roller-coaster. In addition, excess glucagon hormone that is a result of this roller-coaster activity, tends to break down muscles to scavenge for fuels in order to raise blood sugar. That process causes muscle loss and weakness.

### Insulin Leads To Fat Accumulation And Water Retention

High insulin levels not only lead to fat accumulation, but also salt and water retention, which makes you feel bloated and adds pounds. When this happens, insulin stimulates your appetite making you feel hungry. Because the insulin is not working properly, the cells are starving and screaming for more sugar as fuel. That's why you get trapped in a cycle of carbohydrate cravings.

### Healthy Insulin Levels Increase Life

Insulin levels are probably one of the best markers of longevity. When scientists have looked for clues to longevity and studied people who have lived to be over 100, they have found only three common characteristics: low to normal blood sugar, low insulin levels and low HDL (good) cholesterol. That is just another reason why it is important to keep insulin balanced.

### Can I Be Addicted To Sugar?

ABSOLUTELY! Although most people feel satisfaction after eating sugar items or carbohydrates that create sugar in the body, the mechanism is complex. This is because sugar stimulates insulin and insulin serves to transport the amino acid "tryptophan" to the brain where it is used in the production of "serotonin". Serotonin is sometimes referred to as the "feel good chemical" because, when it is elevated, it makes you feel self-confident, calm, composed and generally satisfied. When serotonin levels decline, you feel anxious and depressed. When tryptophan is scarce, serotonin is in short supply. This is an intolerable condition for your brain which demands immediate action. We never want to feel unhappy if we can help it and that's why we experience a craving for sugar.

### Sugar Acts As An Antidepressant

When sugar, in any of its many forms, delivers tryptophan to the brain and restores serotonin levels so you feel happy and generally satisfied, it acts like an antidepressant. In fact, prescription antidepressants work by elevating the level of serotonin in the brain too. Just remember, the brisk swings in blood sugar-insulin-serotonin only temporarily correct low serotonin and hormone imbalance when it's being achieved by too much starch and sugar consumption. What is really needed is multiple amino acids from proteins for stability. When people substitute carbohydrates for protein, they do not have adequate amino acids in their system to build all the neurotransmitters (serotonin, norephinephrine, dopamine, and endorphins) that are required to maintain a healthy balance in the body. Eating protein instead of carbs doesn't stop you from feeling good, it stops the "crash" that makes you eat more of the wrong foods in order to feel better.

More important than simply using food to address an overweight condition, poor nutrition will cause mental changes, depression and agitation all on their own. It is not only the amino acids from protein that are essential, but also the numerous vitamins, minerals, and essential fatty acids that are responsible for regulating optimal brain function and ultimately, physical control. It is important to be aware that so much of what you feel is caused and perpetuated by the food you eat. Mood swings and depression can be greatly controlled by a change in your diet. Sugar creates a negative cycle that is hard to break. Your body's reaction and addiction to the sugar it craves creates your need to eat more in order to feel better.

## WHY AND HOW YOU CORRECT SUGAR IMBALANCES

Insulin levels are mainly determined by sugar and carbohydrates. Protein has a minor effect. When you limit your carbohydrate intake, you stabilize both insulin and glucose levels. Diet is the primary way to control insulin. Exercise will also help control blood sugar fluctuations which, in turn, helps control insulin levels. When weight loss is your goal, be aware that it is impossible without balancing insulin hormone levels. To that end, your diet must be high in protein, low in carbohydrates. Nutritional supplementation in the form of protein shakes and vitamins will also make insulin balance easier. Evaluating your eating patterns should give you an indication of your relationship with sugar:

1. Do you eat regular meals at regular times?
2. Do you snack often?
3. What kind of foods do you eat at meals? Meats? Eggs? Fish? Beans?
4. What snacks do you eat? Crackers? Fruits? Candy? Protein bars/shakes?
5. Do you eat adequate protein daily?
6. How big is each protein portion? 4 oz? 6 oz? 8 oz? 10 oz?
7. How is your food prepared? Breaded? Fried? Grilled? Baked?
8. Do you eat sweets every day?
9. How often do you have dessert?
10. Do you drink soft drinks? Sugar-free? Regular?
11. Do you drink coffee? Coffee beverages, cappuccino?
12. What happens if you do not eat any sugar for 24 hours?

What Do Your Potential Responses Mean?
(Definitions are given by corresponding number)

1. If you don't eat regular meals at regular times, you are creating insulin spikes and irregularity in your body.
2. If you snack often, you are probably not eating balanced meals which creates the need for additional snacks.
3. The kind of foods you eat indicates if your menus are protein or carbohydrate based. Carbohydrates will greatly and negatively impact your insulin levels.
4. The snacks you eat indicate if you have sugar cravings.
5. Eating adequate protein daily insures better insulin health.
6. Your protein portions should not be less that 6 ounces per meal with an over all daily minimum consumption of 10 ounces or 70 grams.
7. If you are breading or frying your foods, you are increasing sugar and fat intake.
8. Eating sweets every day indicates a sugar addiction.
9. How often you eat dessert also indicates the potential for a sugar addiction.
10. Soft drinks are full of sugar. Drinking 'sugar free' soft drinks only stimulates your need and taste for sugar because sugar substitutes are often times sweeter than sugar.
11. Caffeinated beverages can stimulate sweet urges and insulin imbalances.
12. If you get headaches, are irritable or feel nervous when you have not had sugar within 24 hours, you may have a sugar addiction which indicates an insulin problem.

If you have answered these questions honestly, you will be able to identify any problems you might have with the amount of sugar or sugar-producing foods you are currently eating. Unless those problems are addressed, you will be a candidate for diabetes or other sugar-related diseases. You can also look for "hidden sugars" in the chemical synonyms of the foods you eat and try to avoid eating foods containing:

| | | | |
|---|---|---|---|
| * Dextrose | * Glucose | * Fructose | * Corn sweetener |
| * Maltodextrin | * Malt | * Sorghym | * Sucrose |
| * Sorbitol | * Dextrin | * Lactose | * Maltose |
| * Mannitol | * Zylitol | * Modified cornstarch | |
| * Fruit juice concentrates | | * High-fructose corn syrup | |

These are all fancy names for sugar additives. Read product labels and stay away from these ingredients whenever possible.

# 7 DAY PREP: Rebalance Your Hormones

This is a one-week eating plan to get your hormones back in balance. The changes you will make to your current way of eating will be an on-going process. However, the 7-Day Starter will get your body prepared for weight loss. Once your hormones are in balance, cravings and continual hunger will no longer occur. Changing from being a "sugar burner" that continually stores body fat into a "fat burner" who rebuilds lean muscle through proper hormone balance takes about seven days.

Your commitment to the next seven days will determine your future success. The way you need to eat during this time is only TEMPORARY. After seven days, when your hormones are in balance, you will advance to a much simpler and liberal food plan. But, in order to get your body's insulin hormone stabilized, you will need to restrict your carbohydrate and sugar intake greatly the first week.

## *FOR 7 DAYS ONLY*

- ◆ Limit starchy carbohydrates (breads, rice, pasta, potato) to a single serving (approximately 20 grams) per day
- ◆ Eat unlimited protein: seafood, chicken, turkey, beef, pork, eggs, soy products
- ◆ 2 protein shakes count as your starchy carbohydrate serving for the day
- ◆ You may have hard cheeses, low fat cottage cheese and plain yogurt without fruit
- ◆ Eat unlimited non-starchy green vegetables such as lettuce, spinach, broccoli, asparagus, green peppers, green onions, cucumbers and celery
- ◆ Avoid most fruits. You may have a handful of blueberries OR strawberries OR raspberries OR blackberries once or twice each day
- ◆ Drink eight, 8-ounce glasses of water each day (64 ounces)
- ◆ You may have coffee, tea, iced tea or water. No soda, diet soda, alcohol or juices.
- ◆ Try not to eat after 7:00 PM
- ◆ 5-6 small meals are preferred over 2-3 large ones

By not eating after 7:00 PM, the evening fast period will allow your body to restore your hormones and begin to work in your "fat burner" favor. Please note, this type of eating schedule is superb for type 2 diabetics, almost all of whom have high insulin levels.

By the third and forth day, when your sugar/glycogen stores are depleted, your body will begin to convert to being a "fat burner". By day four, cravings should subside and you will start to feel more energetic and in control. If you experience headaches or fatigue the first four days, it is because your body is going through carbohydrate withdrawal. Simply take aspirin or whatever pain reliever you would usually use for headache discomfort. A protein snack will also help you feel better.

## WHAT'S NEXT?

*The Country Club Diet* is unique, exciting and extremely healthy. After the first rebalancing week, you will be allowed to eat all foods within reason. It is important that you are aware how the time of day you eat plays a big role in the processing of food in your body. Obviously, you need to eat when your schedule dictates and cannot get too caught up trying to unrealistically follow rules of this or any diet. But, by simply understanding the benefits of eating smaller meals more frequently, or minimizing heavy, sugar-laden meals just before bedtime, you can take much better control of your hormone balance and body functions.

Remember, a calorie is not just a calorie. Its effects on your body shape depend upon the hormonal environment, the frequency and time your food is eaten and how foods are combined with other foods. For example if you ate 2000 calories in a 24 hour period, your body would have a completely different hormone response if those calories were consumed in two lunch and dinner meals vs. five smaller meals throughout the day. The more you can spread your dining out from morning to evening, the better.

Ideally, it is also better to eat one category of food at a time because the digestive process for each type of food is different. For example, protein digests slowly where carbohydrates digest much faster. When you eat these two food groups together, the protein slows down digestion which can cause the carbs to ferment and putrefy. When this occurs, it can create all sorts of gastrointestinal distress. On the hormonal front, the combination of high carbs and high fat will lead to a high insulin situation whereby most of the absorbed nutrients will go directly to fat storage. That's why, whenever possible, it is better to eat meats with vegetables and without starches. We certainly recognize that this suggestion can be difficult to implement. Do not concern yourself too much if it poses too great a problem for you. We tell you these things so you have more knowledge about how your body works. Being aware will help you make better meal-planning decisions in the future.

The best health programs do not come with "rules" that are difficult to maintain. However, as a starting point, I will give you some basic guidelines to get you started. Try to eat by category and avoid calorie counting or weighing portions whenever possible:

- [ ] Eat as much protein (chicken, seafood, turkey, lean red meat) as possible - a minimum of 10 ounces daily.

- [ ] Vegetables are unlimited daily. Eat all colors. Remember that corn is a starch.

- [ ] Citrus fruits like grapefruit, and lemons or apples and cantaloupe can all be eaten daily. You may also have one handful of berries each day. Limit high sugar fruits like watermelon, pineapple, bananas, and oranges to three times per week or every other day.

- [ ] Select 1 meal for the dairy category. This will help control fat intake. If you have eggs for breakfast, don't have cheese for lunch.

- [ ] Eat 2 portions of starchy carbohydrates each day such as rice, pasta, potato, corn, or bread. For example, you may have a sandwich for lunch and potato or pasta side dish for dinner. Avoid white starches whenever possible.

- [ ] Drink lots of water

When it comes to serving sizes for carbohydrates like breads, pasta, rice, cereal, etcetera, each person has their own individual serving size in mind. Although we do not want you to count calories or grams on this program, you should be aware that your carb intake should not exceed 70-80 grams per day. That usually equates to what most Americans consider to be two servings. For example, the average bagel is now 4 ½ inches in diameter and delivers 60-70 grams of carbohydrates all by itself, yet most people do not feel they are eating as much as 7 servings in that one item. That is what "supersizing," in fast-food lingo, has done to our way of thinking in America!

Because we do not want you to be preoccupied with food or spend your day calculating the impact of what you're eating by counting, weighing or portioning meals, our goal is for you to eat 2 average-sized carbohydrate servings each day. However, this may take time. Cut back carbohydrates slowly and adjust to the quantity as it is most comfortable for you. Since you have now stabilized your hormones after the 7-Day PREP period and have greatly reduced your starch intake during that time, try not to reintroduce too many carbohydrates back into your daily meal plans.

Do not be concerned initially with the size of your fruit, vegetable or protein portions. Just make sure to eat a balance of food daily. The less complicated you make your food program, the more successful the transition will be.

'Worth It' foods is a term I use when I refer to foods that may have questionable food value or high fat content. If you are considering the consumption of any item that fits this description, be sure it is "worth it". Eating a heavy piece of bread just because it is there does not fall into a 'worth it' category. To be 'worth it', it should be wonderfully delicious and "worth" the added burden it places on your body.

Don't be overly aggressive in your menu planning. You want to make reasonable dietary changes that you can live with forever. Temporary food alterations only means temporary weight loss results. Be responsible about your choices and don't eat things you know are not good for you on a regular basis.

If you attempt to deny yourself, you'll start establishing cravings. We always want what we "can't have," so feel comfortable that everything is on your "can have" list. What will surprise you most, is many of the items you now crave will become a thing of the past. Like your body, your taste buds have a memory. Soon you will begin to crave foods that are good for you and never miss the unhealthy staples of your former self.

# FIVE EASY-TO-FOLLOW STEPS

**1.  Stop Dieting And Eat Realistically.**  Do not make drastic food changes that you cannot maintain long term.  You must take an honest look at what and how you eat and evaluate your problem food areas.  Sweets, cheeses and snack foods are obvious areas that can most likely be adjusted.  There is no advantage to eliminating items from your daily menu while trying to lose weight if you intend to eat those items once you have achieved your weight loss goal.  It is not hard to retrain your taste buds and learn to enjoy the foods that are best for you.

**2.  Food Rotation.**  This is the single biggest thing you can do daily to affect your body's metabolism.  Even if you did not change one thing in your regular diet but never ate the same items two days in a row, you would see a weight decrease. If you eat the same foods every day (and most of us do), you are slowing down your metabolism by putting it into a regular pattern.  This is counter-productive.

Rotate all your foods every 24 hours.  If you eat chicken on Monday, do not have it again until Wednesday.  This rule applies to everything you eat, even if those things do not have any calories.  Lettuce is an excellent example.  If you eat iceberg lettuce on Monday, have bibb lettuce on Tuesday and romaine on Wednesday.  The change will keep your metabolic level much more active and your body functioning more efficiently.

**3.  Drink Water.**  Water is the only liquid you can drink that will flush fats out of your body.  Water beverages such as coffee or tea are not water.  Soda is not water.  You must drink six to eight 8-ounce glasses of water daily to eliminate the fats your body is breaking down.  If you do not like water, try some of the flavored waters now available like Syfo or Perrier.

Check the label before you purchase bottled water.  Be sure the label says "0 calories" and no artificial sweeteners.  A lot of "water beverages" now available have as many or more calories than soda and are not water even though the label clearly states "water beverage".  The word "beverage" is a tip off that you are not getting pure water. It is also interesting to note that you will drink two to three times more water if you drink through a straw rather than from a glass.

**4.  Food Trading.**  Many food alternatives, high in protein or low in fat calories, can be substituted for food containing less desirable characteristics.  Once educated about alternative foods, it is a lot easier to make smart choices.  Grate your cheese, don't slice it. You will trick your mind into thinking you are eating a larger quantity. Try eating turkey bacon instead of pork. Eat sugar-free popsicles or frozen yogurt instead of ice cream. Eat fat free pretzels not chips. At any level, for any kind of food category, there is an alternative that is both satisfying and better for you.

**5. Don't Deny Yourself.** This is probably the most important step. No matter what food item you crave, be sure to include a serving or two in your meal planning for the week. It is true that you cannot live on chocolate cake, but you can plan on having a reasonably sized piece once or twice a week and give yourself a treat to look forward to. Find a comfortable eating plan that allows you all the things you like regularly, not necessarily daily, and maintain this pattern forever. If you deny yourself your favorite foods, you will eventually begin to binge on those items until you have satisfied your body's craving.

Be realistic about what you can and cannot live with. This is true of what you eat and also how active you intend to be. Statistics show that more than seventy percent of Americans do not exercise. If you are one of these people, your diet must consist of high protein foods like purltry, seafood and lean red meats rather than heavy carbohydrates such as bread, pasta, rice or potato.

Without extensive exercise, you have no way to burn off the sugar unused carbohydrates produce in order to create energy in your body. That sugar, or glucose, is what your body will ultimately turn into fat. When you consider it takes fifteen minutes of jogging for your body to burn off a single slice of bread, you need to evaluate your carbohydrate consumption in relation to your activity level.

## FOCUS ON PROTEIN

Protein is essential for growth and development. It is part of every living cell and makes up tissue, skin, bone, hair, blood and muscle. It is critical for both balanced health and weight management. Since protein is not stored in the body like carbohydrates or fats, each person needs to regularly replenish an adequate supply. There are many theories about how much protein should be consumed daily. According to the US government, the average person should eat about 70 grams of protein each day which equates to approximately 10 ounces of poultry, seafood or lean red meat. Some experts feel at least 1 gram of protein should be eaten daily for each pound of body weight. Keeping the 10 ounce number as a minimum requirement, try to eat as much protein as you can.

At least half of the protein you eat is burned up in the digestive process. Protein has the ability to stimulate the metabolism through it's thermogenic or 'fat burning' effect and stabilizes insulin levels which is needed in order to metabolize fat properly. In addition, it provides the body with:

- Energy and heat
- Contributes to the composition of the body's fluids
- Transports substances through the blood stream
- Helps maintain proper acid-alkali balance
- Builds new body tissues and repairs damaged ones
- Helps build resistance to disease in the formation of antibodies
- Needed for the manufacture and building of hormones, antibodies and enzymes

When protein is consumed, the body breaks it down into amino acids which are the building blocks of all proteins. There are 22 necessary amino acids. Some of the amino acids are designated "non-essential". This does not mean that they are unnecessary, but rather that they do not have to come from the diet because they can be synthesized by the body from other amino acids already housed there. Additionally, some amino acids are considered "essential", meaning that the body cannot make them by itself and must obtain them from food sources or protein supplements.

Whenever the body makes a protein, it needs a variety of amino acids for the protein-making process. These amino acids may come from dietary protein or from the body's own pool of amino acids.

### *The Effects Of A Low-Protein Diet*

If your diet is deficient in high protein foods containing essential amino acids, the building of protein in your body stops. When this occurs:

- Cells cannot function properly
- Cellular repair is handicapped
- Immune function is impaired
- Irregularities in body functions occur
- You are more susceptible to disease

Additionally, if your diet is protein deficient, your body could also be deficient in many important vitamins and minerals found in protein-rich foods. Niacin, thiamin, riboflavin, B-12, B-6, iron, zinc and calcium, among others, are best obtained from protein-rich food sources. What we eat creates a chain effect. When you fail to eat adequate supplies of one food group, it will affect the necessary nutrients that your body needs that are housed within that group. In many instances, nutrients from one food group help the body absorb necessary nutrients from another. That is why it is so important to eat a well-balanced food plan.

## PROTEIN SOURCES

There is a wide variety of protein sources available. Some have higher fat content than others. Protein powders also provide a complete source of protein and can do so without the additional associated fat or calories found in traditional protein foods. If you are eating protein supplements, however, make sure you select a brand that provides you with a complete amino acid complex in order to maximize the protein you are eating and is not full of carbohydrates.

Good sources of protein are:

- Beef
- Lamb
- Seafood
- Cheese
- Pork
- Chicken
- Tofu
- Vegetarian proteins
- Liver
- Turkey
- Soy
- Veal
- Duck
- Eggs

Although it is important for you to eat the full range of essential and non-essential amino acids every day, it is not necessary to get them from meat, fish, poultry, and other complete protein foods. Vegetable proteins, when combined properly, can form a complete protein that is a high quality substitute for meat. For example, beans and brown rice are both quite rich in protein but, individually, each lacks one or more of the necessary amino acids. Combined together in a meal, they create a perfect or complete protein.

### How Does A Vegetarian Eat Enough Protein?

There are all kinds of vegetarians. Some eat chicken and fish, others stay away from any animal products including milk or cheese. Depending upon which kind of vegetarian you may be, our best advise is to go to the local bookstore to pick up a vegetarian cookbook. Many cookbooks will include the nutritional information for each recipe including protein, approximate fat and carbohydrate content. Since creating proteins with the combination of beans and rice can be like conducting a scientific experiment, we urge you to find the foods that are most interesting to you and build your menus around those. Tofu, for example, is an excellent source of protein. But, this may or may not be an acceptable alternative for your personal taste buds.

To make your understanding a little easier, here's a list of vegetarian proteins that may be helpful in your quest for 70 - 100 grams of protein each day:

## Low Fat Proteins

| | |
|---|---|
| ½ cup cottage cheese | 12 grams |
| 1 meatless burger | 12 grams |
| 1 cup wild rice | 12 grams |
| 8 oz. low fat yogurt | 9-12 grams |
| 3 egg whites | 11 grams |
| ½ cup soft tofu | 10 grams |
| 1 cup milk | 8 grams |
| 1 cup brown rice | 6 grams |
| ½ cup legumes, black beans, kidney beans, lentils and split peas | 6 grams |

## High Fat Proteins

| | |
|---|---|
| ½ cup firm tofu | 20 grams |
| 1 oz. mozzarella cheese | 6 grams |
| 1 oz. cheddar cheese | 7 grams |
| 1 oz. American cheese | 6 grams |
| 1 oz. peanuts | 7 grams |
| 10 oz. sunflower seeds | 7 grams |
| 10 oz. almonds | 6 grams |
| 2 tablespoons peanut butter | 8 grams |

*Complete Proteins When Mixed Together*

Rice & beans

Rice & lentils

*Fat-Free Processed Items Are Not Good Protein Sources*

Many people assume that fat-free or even low-fat dairy items should be considered a protein because there is no longer fat in the item. Not so. In the event that fat has been removed from a food, that fat is generally replaced with sugar or carbohydrates to retain its taste. Fat by itself does not make you fat. Nuts, for example, are full of fat. However, they contain essential fatty acid fats that are very beneficial to your body. They come from nature and have not been manipulated by man. Those cannot be confused with the manufactured fats that are added into man-made, processed foods. Do not be lulled into eating "fat free" foods thinking you are making a smarter choice. Fat free dairy, like yogurt or skim milk, have high carbohydrate content and will raise insulin levels that will subsequently cause the glucose those foods are creating to be stored as fat. You are much better off eating dairy items in the natural way they were intended to be eaten… fat and all!

# CARBOHYDRATES

There are two types of carbohydrates: Simple and Complex. The physical properties of carbohydrates cause them to be digested at different rates. The quicker the rate of digestion, the greater the rise in blood sugar and increased negative impact on the body.

**Simple Carbohydrates** are sugars like table sugar, candy, cookies, etcetera.

**Complex Carbohydrates** are grains, legumes, fruits, vegetables and starches. As a food group, starchy carbohydrates have the most negative impact on your body. They are the quickest to digest and cause insulin levels to climb. They are found in foods like breads, pasta, rice, potato, corn, chips, crackers or cereal as well as dried fruit, fruit juice and soda.

These kinds of starchy foods are the most dangerous of all carbohydrates because, in order to create energy, the starches consumed turn into glucose or sugar. When you do not expend enough energy daily to burn up the excess glucose created, the sugar produced by these foods is stored and ultimately turns to fat. Even eating low fat or fat-free starches won't help you avoid the body's own fat manufacturing that goes with carbohydrate consumption. The fat that starch causes your body to make is a result of the high sugar production those carbohydrates create.

Eating a high carbohydrate, low protein, low fat diet will result in excess fat storage. You will find you are craving more starches or sweets with great regularity. You will have low energy, mood swings and constant hunger while your metabolism slows and does not burn fat efficiently. As a healthy alternative, using protein for energy allows your body to keep your insulin levels low which burns more fat. Fat provides more than twice the energy of carbohydrates. One way to determine if you are eating too many carbohydrates is to evaluate if you are able to go four hours without eating. If not, chances are that your starchy carbohydrate intake is too high.

It takes 15 minutes of jogging for the body to burn off a single slice of bread. We encourage you to eat a balanced diet that includes all food groups, but carbohydrates should be minimized. Avoid white starches as much as possible. White potatoes, white rice, sugar frosted cereals, white bread, white pasta, French fries, all have high sugar content with little or no nutritional value. As a matter of fact, a baked potato has the sugar equivalent of a piece of chocolate cake! When you think of it that way, why waste your 'dessert' on a baked potato?

As a nutritional rule of thumb, minimize white starches. That does not mean you cannot enjoy these kinds of food altogether. It simply means you should eat healthier versions of the same item. Try whole grain breads like wheat or rye instead of white bread... eat a sweet potato instead of a white potato... try spinach pasta instead of enriched flour pasta... select whole grain or wild rice instead of white rice. It will not take long for you to retrain your taste buds to prefer foods that are better for you. Most of the "alternative" suggestions we have made have much more flavor than their white counterpart. Spices also make a big difference. Season your foods well and you will enjoy them more. The act of eating isn't generally about what goes into your stomach as much as it is about how that food tastes. Be creative. You can make anything taste good if you simply set your mind to it.

# THINK "NET CARBS"

You can increase your daily carbohydrate consumption if you select carbs that have a high fiber content. Since fiber is so important for proper maintenance of the body through its cleansing properties, you can actually deduct the fiber content contained in a carbohydrate food to get the 'net carb' impact of that item. For example, if you eat a whole wheat English muffin that contains 44 grams of carbohydrate and 7 grams of fiber, the net carb result of that English muffin would be 37 net carbohydrates.

People sometimes get confused about vegetables and even avoid eating them because many are high in complex carbohydrates. Don't be confused! Vegetables are an important addition to meals. They are high in fiber and should be eaten regularly. A whole bunch of broccoli (approximately 8 cups!) contains 40 grams of carbohydrate and 16 grams of fiber which makes the net carb result only 24. Obviously, a person would get VERY full eating 8 cups of broccoli so you can see how you can maximize the carbohydrates you eat if you think ahead and plan.

Almonds and nuts are another item that can make a terrific snack with a low net carbohydrate impact. 1 ounce of almonds has 5 grams of carbohydrate and 3 grams of fiber making a net carb result of only 2 grams. Plus, you get essential fatty acids in almonds along with 6 grams of protein making almonds a great food item.

As a basic rule of thumb, you want to limit your carbohydrate intake to approximately 70 NET grams per day so read the labels on the products you buy. Most fruits & vegetables are usually pretty high in fiber so you need not worry about the carb impact of those foods. We don't want you to count calories or weigh portions, but we do want you to become aware of smarter food choices. Even items like yogurt can be very high in carbohydrates. We know of one brand that contains more than 40 carbs in a single serving along with more sugar than a soda! Once identified, that would be a product to avoid. You don't need to be afraid of carbs, you simply need to be smart about the ones you select.

# MEAL SKIPPING AND THE IMPORTANCE OF BREAKFAST

Numerous studies have proven the benefits on body shape and fat composition when people eat frequent, smaller meals rather than two or three large ones each day. It is not only the amount or type of food you eat that is important, it is the frequency of your food intake that ultimately determines your body's health, weight and contour.

Frequent, smaller meals have many physical advantages for your body:

- It is easier for the body to process smaller amounts of food at a time, making it operate more efficiently.
- Frequent, smaller meals lead to a lower overall insulin response, there fore allowing more fat burning which prevents your body from going into a fat storage mode.
- It keeps the metabolic rate higher. Your body will continue working rather than shut down between the fewer vs. larger portions being consumed. Food, (especially protein which is very thermogenic) is the fuel needed to stoke your metabolic furnace.
- Regular meals help control cravings and eliminate severe hunger drives that may lead to overeating.
- Regular meals encourage fat usage and preserves muscle-mass.
- Regular meals keep cortisol excretion lower. Cortisol is the stress hormone that tends to break down muscle tissue and causes insulin resistance, abdominal obesity and numerous other harmful effects.

Meal skipping puts your body into hormonal and metabolic chaos, which prevents weight loss. In the morning, your body has been without food for 8-12 hours which creates a decreased metabolic rate and fat hoarding. Breakfast is needed to jump-start the day's metabolic processes. A good breakfast, which includes adequate protein, will increase your metabolic rate at least 10%. It keeps your body balanced both hormonally and metabolically and will ward off energy crashes, hypoglycemia, cravings and binges. When you skip breakfast, even if you are not hungry in the morning, it causes your metabolic system to slow while increasing hunger. This practice generally leads to overeating at lunch too.

So, what should you eat? Traditional breakfast foods like bacon, cereal, pancakes or waffles are not adequate sources of protein. Additionally, eating high carbohydrate items such as toast or cereal will send insulin levels soaring, leaving you hungry again by ten or eleven in the morning. Ideal breakfast fare should be high in protein like protein shakes, eggs, salmon or other fish, yogurt, breakfast steaks, dinner meats and vegetable leftovers. You may need to develop a new way of thinking when it comes to breakfast food fare.

## Eating By Category

To make meal planning simple and avoid counting calories, know that you can eat unlimited proteins, fruits and vegetables every day. In order to minimize fats, limit the amount of dairy you eat to one or two servings. If the dairy item you select is fat-free, then you may consider that a carbohydrate. Remember, when fats are removed, sugar or carbohydrates are usually substituted in order for the food item to retain its flavor.

Starchy carbohydrates should be capped at two to three servings daily. If you are having a sandwich at lunch, then you may have a sweet potato, brown rice or a side of pasta for dinner. It is always best to make your starches a side dish rather than an entrée. This trick will also ensure that you are eating enough protein. If you fill up on meats, fruits and vegetables, you will have much less room for the sugars and starches you are trying to minimize.

Our goal is for you to feel full, not hungry. When you eat by category and do not weigh, sort, plan and count calories every day, you will take a lot of your focus off food. Overweight people have a tendency to think about food a lot. It's important that you don't put yourself on a "diet" with all the restrictions dieting implies. Even eating by category allows you to eat anything you want. It simply doesn't let you eat everything you want all the time. You will simply need to learn how to make responsible choices about the foods you select. Your body deserves that consideration.

## Timing Is Everything

If you think of your body as a cycling machine, it will help you to understand why the timing of your meals are important. We certainly understand that it may not be possible for you to eat in this recommended manner. However, it is the optimum way in which you can be sure your body burns more fat and is able to lose weight the fastest. It is important that you create an eating plan for yourself that fits realistically into your lifestyle. But, the more aware you are of the advantages of eating early in the day, the better able you are to adjust meal times where adjustments are possible.

In an ideal world, without outside influences to alter schedules, the perfect way to eat would be as follows:

**Breakfast:** For all the reasons previously mentioned, breakfast is the meal that gets your body's engine started and pumps the metabolism. If you really want to eat carbohydrates, this is the meal to do it. But, you need to include an adequate amount of protein too. Eggs, salmon, breakfast steak and even leftovers all make a great breakfast. Remember, if you are eating carbohydrates for this meal, stick with whole grains and avoid white starches.

Use your handful of berries as a snack or eat them with breakfast or lunch. Avoid any fruit after 6:PM in the evening. The sugar content in fruit will elevate insulin production and slow fat burn.

**Lunch & Dinner:** Keep meals lean with lots of protein and vegetables. Your second starch of the day is best eaten at lunch if possible.

For best weight loss results: Do not eat ANYTHING after 7:00 in the evening. The majority of your food should be consumed during your high activity, daytime hours. After 7:PM, your body is preparing for rest. Eating food after this hour increases insulin production which interrupts fat burn and repair cycles. Fat loss will be much faster if you do not consume any food after 7:00 in the evening. You may drink water.

# FOOD CATEGORIES

The following list of foods in each of the food groups will help you better understand the options you have. If a food is not listed, it does not mean that it should be avoided. We have simply covered only the basics here.

**PROTEIN**
**Seafood - Low fat**
**Unlimited Daily**

Cod
Crab
Flounder
Grouper
Haddock
Halibut
Lobster
Salmon
Scallops
Scrod
Sole
Shrimp
Swordfish
Tuna Fish (water packed)
Whitefish
Dolphin

**Meat - Low Fat**
**Unlimited Daily**

Beef Liver
Chicken
Chicken Liver
Turkey

**Meat - High Fat**
**Unlimited Daily**

Club Steak
Flank Steak
Filet Mignon
Ground Turkey
Ground Sirloin
Lamb Chops
London Broil
Prime Rib
Roast Beef
Veal

**VEGETABLES**
**Unlimited Daily**

Asparagus
Bean Sprouts
Cabbage
Carrots
Cauliflower
Celery
Cucumber
Eggplant
Green Beans
Lettuce - all varieties
Mushrooms
Onions
Peppers
Radishes
Spinach
Squash
Tomatoes
Zucchini

**FRUITS**
**Low Sugar**
**Unlimited**

Apples
Cantaloupe
Grapefruit
Lemons

**Higher Sugar**
**3X Per Week**

Apricots
Bananas
Honeydew
Nectarine
Orange
Papaya
Peach
Pear & Plum
Pineapple
Tangerine
Watermelon

**Avoid All Dried Fruit**
**& Cranberry Sauce**

**VEGETARIAN**
**Limited - 3X Per Week**
**Vegetarians Only**
Boca Burgers
Tofu
Soy Milk
Veggie Burgers

**DAIRY - FATS**
**1 Serving Daily**

Butter
Cheese
Cream Cheese
Cottage Cheese
Eggs
Mayonnaise
Milk
Parmesan Cheese
Yogurt

**STARCHES**
**2 Servings Daily**

Bread
Bagel (Scooped)
Bialy
Cereal (Hot or Cold)
Crackers
Pancakes/Waffles
Pasta
Peas
Pita Bread
Potato
Rice
Tortillas

**Fruit - Berries**
**Limited to 1 Handful Daily**

Blackberries
Blueberries
Cherries
Grapes
Star Fruit
Strawberries

# GLYCEMIC INDEX

The glycemic index is a food ranking system that rates foods relative to how fast they are absorbed into the body and how quickly they raise blood sugar levels. Foods that spike blood sugar levels are called "high glycemic" foods. They also spike insulin to high levels which leads to fat storage.

More important than a food's glycemic index is its GLYCEMIC LOAD. The "load" takes into account the total amount of actual sugar in the food. For example, carrots have a higher glycemic index than M&M candy. However, M&M's have much more sugar per gram weight which leads to a higher insulin level, or "load" than carrots. There are many diets that suggest you select your foods based on their glycemic load. This requires that you use a glycemic index chart and multiply each food's glycemic index by it carbohydrate content in order to calculate its load. We do NOT suggest you do this exercise, but we do want you to be aware of how glycemic index and glycemic load works.

**Foods with a HIGH glycemic load cause a greater insulin spike response. The following foods should be minimized and avoided whenever possible:**

| | | | |
|---|---|---|---|
| * white bread | * bagels | * English muffins | * flaked cereals |
| * instant hot cereal | * raisins | * dried fruits | * low-fat frozen desserts |
| * whole milk | * peanuts | * peanut butter | * whole milk cheeses |
| * luncheon meat | * hot dogs | * candy bars | * all refined grains and sugars |

**Foods with a LOW glycemic load are generally higher in fiber and roughage. They are more slowly digested and absorbed in the body which leads to a slow, gradual raise in blood sugar, providing the body with a controlled insulin and hormone response. The following are your most beneficial choices:**

| | | | |
|---|---|---|---|
| * fresh vegetables | * leafy greens | * whole-grain breads | * sweet potatoes |
| * yams | * skim milk | * buttermilk* poultry | * lean beef & pork |
| * veal | * shellfish | * white fish | * most legumes |
| * most nuts | * whole-grain cereal | | |

# Vitamins and Nutritional Tools

It is impossible for you to get all the proper nutrition your body needs daily through food. The food you consume today is not in the league of the food quality produced a half-century ago. Today your body requires nutritional fortification to be healthy. However, unlike years past, your body is further challenged by a tremendous toxic load of food chemicals, pesticides, air pollution, hormones and other additives that breed disease. You cannot fight these elements with food alone.

When you are nutritionally and hormonally imbalanced, weight loss is almost impossible. No amount of dieting or exercise will get you to your goal weight if your body is blocking your progress.

We live in a very toxic environment. Poor food choices and a diet full of sugar and refined carbohydrates generate more toxins. These can be just as poisonous to the body as industrial chemicals. Remember, government statistics indicate that you are consuming approximately twenty pounds of chemicals and food additives each year and as much as forty pounds if fast, frozen or convenience foods are a regular part of your diet. Your metabolic problems, hormone conditions, diseases and aging are all caused by cumulative free-radical damage. A high quality daily multi-vitamin and antioxidant are critical in order for you to optimize your metabolism and maximally support the health and energy production of every cell in your body in order to make weight loss possible. When you are nutritionally imbalanced, your body will retain stored body fat, rather than burn it. It does this in order to protect its vital organs. Unless you provide your body with the nutrition it requires, your body will not release fat, no matter what you do.

Many food additives can cause your body to misidentify foods and process them through the system inefficiently. Your immune system is greatly challenged because it cannot detoxify these elements from the foods you are eating fast enough. Many of these foreign chemicals slip through and float directly into your blood stream as if you have a virus or other kind of bacteria in your system. Your body may respond to this chemical insult in any number of physical ailments such as irritable bowel syndrome, chronic headache, fatigue, or stomach problems. In addition, the edge may be taken off of your athletic performance and you may experience an increase in muscle weakness or even inflammation of joints.

Vitamins and nutritional tools in the form of supplements are an excellent means for you to get the nutrition you need without overeating. They will improve your mental and physical response to stress while reducing the body's aches and pains. Proper supplementation can help give your skin a more healthy appearance, protect your body from environmental pollutants and allow important nutrients to be absorbed throughout your body, right down to the cellular level. But, it is important that you take products that are designed to work together rather than self-medicate with a variety of non-related items off local health store shelves. Vitamins and other supplements can also be toxic when taken incorrectly or if their ingredients are not in harmony with one another, so it is important to seek knowledgeable guidance when developing a personal nutritional supplement program.

Never take a vitamin or antioxidant on an empty stomach. They should always be taken with food or your body will be unable to absorb them. In addition, it is best if they are taken twice daily, approximately 10-12 hours apart, so you can maintain 24-hour nutritional protection. Most of your body's healing and repair are done while you are sleeping. If you take all your supplements in the morning, your body does not have the adequate nutritional support necessary to properly heal and rebuild itself.

Protein supplements are also important every day because protein is essential for your body to be able to build muscle, joints, bones, enzymes, hormones, blood cells, healthy skin, hair, nails and all other tissues. Your body cannot store protein so you need a constant supply in order to repair, heal, and regenerate cells and tissues. Taking a protein supplement in the form of a shake or bar can provide your body with a significant number of concentrated proteins without the fat, calories or additional hormones and additives associated with meat products.

Be sure to find protein supplements that are high in protein and low in carbohydrate. Many commercial protein supplements are promoted as meal replacements and are designed to fill you up by including 20-35 grams of carbohydrates per serving in their formulation. This kind of protein supplement should NOT be taken in association with a meal since it is a meal replacement.

If you are going to eat carbohydrate servings with your meals, you do not want to double up by eating full servings of carbohydrates in your protein supplements. For best fortification, protein supplements should be low in carbohydrates and taken in addition to meals and not as a replacement for them.

# EATING ORGANIC

In order for a food to be termed "organic," it must be produced without pesticides, toxic fertilizers, bioengineering or ionizing radiation. Organic meat, poultry, eggs and dairy products must come from animals that are given no antibiotics or growth hormones to fatten them up. Before a product can be labeled "organic," an inspector visits the farm where the food is produced to make sure the farm meets USDA standards. A food must be no less than 95% "organically clean" in order to carry an official "USDA Organic" seal.

Because of the stringent regulations now posed on farmers of organic items, studies have shown that the nutritional quality of the fruits and vegetables grown under these standards are significantly higher than their 'supermarket food' counterpart. Part of the explanation for this is the simple fact that many of the chemicals and fertilizers used in commercial farming leaches soil of important nutrients. Consequently, those nutrients become deficient in foods historically containing them. For example, a governmental study concluded that organic apples, pears, potatoes and wheat had, on an average, 90% more of the expected nutritional elements than their commercially grown counterparts.

What does that mean to you? Simple. Eating "organic" will provide you with a much higher source of nutrition and much lower exposure to dangerous, toxic chemicals. Pesticides in foods are real and they do cause physical harm. The liver is your body's main detoxifying organ and it can be stressed from exposure to the vast variety of chemicals used. When overstressed it will not work well enough to neutralize poisonous invaders so many of the side effects of these toxic chemicals are not metabolized out of your body. They also become a major source of disease which is introduced to you through food and water. Pesticides have been known to increase breast cancer risk, Parkinson's, Gehrigs Disease and can cause thyroid damage which affects everything from weight to mood.

The American public is taking a much closer look at their own personal health. There is no question that your body will benefit from minimizing unnecessary chemicals, toxins or hormones found in non-organic foods. But, in order to be as protective of what you eat as you would like, READ THE LABELS! Food producers are smart and know the public will pay more for organic foods. That's why they will mix organic ingredients with non-organic ones, then promote the organic ingredients prominently on the packaging. Now, with new legislation, you can rest assured that an item must be at least 70% organic in order to significantly promote it as such. Just be sure you are not purchasing "organic junk food" that may be safe from a chemical perspective, but is still full of sugar and other undesirable ingredients that do not provide any nutritional value to you whatsoever.

Free range beef and chicken do not have estrogens, artificial hormones, antibiotics or pesticides in their meat and are well worth the extra expense. When animals are free range, they eat grass and have a higher amount of omega 3 fatty acids in their meat than when the animal is corn fed.

Farm-raised fish should also be avoided if possible. Farm raised salmon has become an abundant commodity. Grown in giant pens, this fish, which lacks government labeling to notify you of its potential health dangers, is subject to contamination from antibiotics, exposed to pesticides, chemicals and has most likely been dyed with color additives. Fish farmers feed synthetic pigment to salmon in order to maintain a pretty pink color. Although affordable and available year-round, farm raised salmon can be detrimental to your health.

Industrial fish farming has experts concerned about the chemicals and pollutants that are damaging the marine environment. Highly concentrated protein fish feeds, fish waste and uneaten food are generating bacteria on these farms that consume oxygen vital to shellfish and other bottom-dwelling sea animals living on the ocean floor. Disease and parasites, which are usually rare in wild, free-swimming fish, abound in fish that are raised in such confined conditions. Typical salmon farms are 100 feet square and will house 50,000-90,000 fish!

Tons of fish died in 2002 due to toxic algae and many had to be destroyed because they carried infectious viruses. None of this requires disclosure to the public on product labeling in the form of warnings so you can make knowledgeable supermarket purchases. Farm salmon are much fattier than wild salmon yet they contain much fewer beneficial omega-3 fatty acids. They also contain much higher quantities of mercury.

Many local markets now carry organic foods. Commercial markets are increasing their organic options and growing national chains like Whole Foods, which carries just about everything from fruits and vegetables to free range chickens and beef in organic form. But, take note... organic foods cost more. If you cannot afford to buy organic fruits and vegetables, non-organic fresh produce is better than not eating fruits and vegetables at all. Fresh produce and butcher-shop items are a necessary part of a good, balanced eating plan. Stay away from canned, boxed or packaged food whenever possible. That's where preservatives and extra fat and chemicals abound. The closer to nature your food is, the better it is for you.

# WATER AFFECTS YOUR HEALTH

Incredible as it may seem, water is quite possibly the single most important ingredient for maintaining a healthy body as well as losing weight and keeping it off. Water flushes fat and toxins from your body, suppresses your appetite naturally and helps your body metabolize stored fat, which means water helps flush fat away. Studies have shown that a decrease in water intake will cause fat deposits to increase, while an increase in water intake can actually reduce fat deposits.

**Water is the best treatment for fluid retention too.** When your body gets less water, it perceives this as a threat to survival and begins to hold onto every available drop it can store. Water is stored in extra-cellular spaces outside the cells which appears to you and me as swollen feet, legs and hands. Diuretics offer a temporary solution at best. They force out stored water along with some essential nutrients. Again, your body perceives a health threat when you don't drink enough water and will replace the lost water at its first opportunity so the 'swollen feet' condition will quickly return.

**Water helps to maintain proper muscle tone** by giving muscles their natural ability to contract while preventing dehydration. It also helps to prevent sagging skin that usually follows weight loss. While water is flushing out fats, it is also flushing out toxins... the same toxins that can carry disease or cause acne and other skin outbreaks. Shrinking cells are buoyed by water, which plumps the skin and leaves it clear, healthy and resilient.

**Water helps rid your body of waste.** During weight loss periods, your body has a lot more waste to dispose. All metabolized fat that has been broken down and is ready to be eliminated must be eliminated from your body through urination. Water will also help relieve constipation. When you do not drink enough water, your body will look to other sources like the colon for hydration. When the colon becomes too dry, you will become constipated and have difficulty going to the bathroom. You can best identify the likelihood of your being dehydrated if you are experiencing thirst, itchy dry skin, fatigue or have headaches.

*A few basic true facts about water:*

- Your body will not function properly without enough water.
- Your body cannot eliminate unwanted, metabolized fat without enough water.
- Retained water in your body is evident through swollen feet and excess weight.
- To eliminate excess water you must drink MORE water!
- Drinking water is essential to weight loss…it is the only way to flush fat from your body.

**How much water is enough?** On the average, you should drink six to eight, 8-ounce glasses every day. That is about two quarts. Seriously overweight or obese people need one additional glass for every 25 pounds of excess weight. Some doctors feel that half your body weight should be consumed in ounces of water daily. In other words, if you weigh 170 lbs., you should drink 85 ounces of water every day. The total amount of water should also be increased if you are exercising or spending a lot of time outdoors where the weather is hot or dry.

Cold water is absorbed into the system more quickly than warm water, but it should not be ice-cold. If you do not like water's flavor, add a squeeze of lemon or lime to your drink. You can also drink your water through a straw or sports bottle. That will actually enable you to consume two to three times more water than you would when drinking from a glass.

Drink spring water rather than tap water whenever possible. The chlorine contained in city drinking water that is used for water purification creates free radicals and can be toxic. Bottled water is much safer and healthier for you to drink.

# WHAT DOES FIBER DO?

As we keep explaining throughout this book, good health and effective weight loss depends upon the coordination of so many parts of your body. A critical function often taken for granted is your intestinal system. For thousands of years, the Chinese, Indians and many schools of Europe believe that the gut is responsible for as much as 70-90% of chronic illnesses. The gastrointestinal tract is associated with 70-75% of the body's defense system. Adequate fiber and nutritional support is required every day to ensure the delicate and harmonious balance with food products, hormones, chemicals and enzymes.

The average diet is deficient in fibrous nutrients. Fruits, vegetables, whole grains and flax are all fibrous cleansing agents that provide numerous important health benefits:

△ Satiety. A sense of having eaten sufficiently.

△ Decreased appetite.

△ Maintenance of weight loss.

△ Lowers blood pressure.

△ Maintains regular bowel. Relieves constipation.

△ Lowers triglycerides, fatty acids and cholesterol in the blood.

△ Slows absorption of sugar thus lowering insulin response.

△ Decreases fat storage.

△ Improves diabetes.

△ Binds and lowers toxins in colon.

△ Decreases incidence of colon cancer.

△ Decreases re-absorption of toxins.

△ Produces short-chained fatty acids which keep the intestinal lining cells healthy.

When your intestinal tract is working efficiently, it is much easier for your body to stay healthy and to lose weight. When it is not, losing weight and weight maintenance becomes quite difficult. With good intestinal health your body decreases the "poison load." Poison load slows or stops the metabolism from working which prevents fat loss. If your body remains in a "toxic state" with the cells surrounded by a poisonous cesspool, then no amount of good nutrition will spark metabolism and weight loss. The bowel must be healthy too.

Imbalance of the intestinal system, specifically the small and large bowel, can cause a wide variety of illnesses and seriously contribute to obesity and weight gain. An intestinal imbalance leads to food cravings, fatigue, depression, anxiety, allergies and headaches. You may not even experience bowel symptoms with an unhealthy GI tract, or you may feel bloated, find yourself regularly constipated, or have diarrhea. This condition will also block proper absorption of important nutrients in your body. If this sounds like you, you are not alone. It is estimated that somewhere between 40 and 80 million people have GI dysfunction.

Many illnesses are related to a "leaky gut" problem which means that the food you eat is not staying and digesting within the stomach and intestine. Partially digested food is escaping into the blood stream through the intestinal walls. The body sees these particles as foreign invaders and mobilizes the immune system to handle them. This condition is so common because poor digestion, enzyme deficiency, numerous prescription drugs like antibiotics and steroids, as well as anti-inflammatory drugs such as ibuprofen can contribute to "leaky gut" syndrome.

If you find you are prone to upset stomach or feel nauseous after eating, you may have a leaky gut. Asthma and other allergies are also indicators. In addition, this disorder is common among children with attention deficit (ADD, ADHD). Treatment of stomach disorders, asthma and other allergies can be greatly improved by addressing the problem with regular cleansing nutrition such as fiber.

For maximal health, energy, vitality, weight loss, and lean body contour, your internal environment must be clean and healthy so energy metabolism and hormonal communications work effectively. Eating adequate fiber helps heal the intestinal lining while restoring intestinal health and normal bacterial balance. As you detoxify your body, you will be better primed for maximum health and weight loss.

## 10 Helpful Hints To Add Fiber And Flavor To Your Diet.

1. Serve meats on top of grains.  Chicken, fish and beef dishes are far more interesting when served on a bed of lentils, barley, couscous or whole-grain rice.

2. Eat citrus fruits, don't juice them.  The white part of the fruit rind is a great source of fiber.  Peel grapefruits and oranges leaving some of the rind in tact. Evidence is mounting that soluble fibers such as those found in apples, peaches, pears, oranges and grapefruits can help lower and may even prevent high cholesterol levels and blood pressure, which reduces the risk of  heart disease and diabetes.

3. Add wheat bran to chicken or seafood breading.  Shaking a 1/2 cup of wheat bran into breading can boost fiber-poor meals without adding a lot of additional calories.

4. Add vegetables to entrée dishes.  Toss broccoli, spinach or peppers onto pizza or mix them with your favorite pasta dish.  Scrambled eggs or omelets take on a new appeal when served 'primavera'.  Try it!

5. Eat high fiber breakfast cereals for snacks.  If you like cereal, have it as a snack instead of a breakfast food.  If you have a hard time sleeping at night, a bowl of cereal rich in high fiber will often do the trick to help you sleep more soundly. Read the label to be sure the cereal you select is not high in sugar and carbohydrates. This is an area where **"net carbs"** is important.

6. Eat sweet potatoes baked, not mashed or fried.  If you must have a baked  white potato, eating it with the skin on is a huge improvement in terms of fiber over a regular potato prepared any other way.  Sweet potatoes are a much better choice because they have much more flavor than a regular potato, provide more nutritional value, have a lower glycemic index and require less condiments.

7.  Make your French toast with whole grain bread.  Whole grain pancake mixes are also available.

8.  Toss a spinach salad.  Plain iceberg lettuce is fairly low in fiber.  If you're not much of a spinach fan, chop the leaves well along with additional fresh vegetables and mix your other lettuce with it.

9. Eat raw vegetables as a snack. Raw vegetables provide the crunch most snackers are looking for and are full of fiber and important nutrients.

10. Chow down on chili. Chili beans are a wonderful source of fiber. When prepared with meat and zesty sauces, it becomes a great source of high protein too. Add canned or cooked chili beans to your favorite stews or soups.

# DON'T COUNT CALORIES... MAKE CALORIES COUNT

What you eat and its nutritional value are far more important than the number of calories that food contains. Eating 1000 calories of chocolate in one day will set your body into an insulin tailspin. Whereas, 1000 calories of chicken will get your fat-burning engines revving. Let's recap the best eating guidelines for an ongoing, healthy lifestyle:

△ Eat whole, fresh, and unprocessed foods as much as possible.

△ Avoid simple or refined carbohydrates (white potato, white bread, white rice, pasta) and sugar products. Replace them with complex carbs such as whole grains, beans, fruits and vegetables. Complex carbohydrates are easier on the pancreas and promote insulin balance. When mixed with fiber, you can eat more

△ Eat at least three regular meals per day. Or, eat five or six smaller meals throughout the day. This helps stabilize the release of blood sugar and insulin.

△ Eat adequate amounts of protein (meat, chicken, fish, eggs, beans, tofu and nuts) at each meal. Proteins take longer to break down in the body thus stabilizing blood sugar levels.

△ Avoid foods made with hydrogenated oils. Be sure to incorporate adequate amounts of healthy fats, such as olive, sesame, or flaxseed oil in your diet. Healthy fats slow the release of sugar into the bloodstream.

△ Reduce intake of fruit juices and dried fruits. Drink vegetable juices and herbal teas instead. Fruit sugars as well as carrot juice can cause a rapid rise in blood sugar levels.

△ Reduce intake of alcohol and caffeinated beverages. Both stimulate blood sugar and insulin.

△ Avoid artificial sweeteners and any products containing them. Sweeteners are both unhealthy and increase your desire for more sweets.

# Be
# A
# Smart
# Consumer

# READ LABELS & COMPARISON SHOP

Most of us purchase the same food products regularly. We tend to buy the same brand names and items without really thinking about it. Take the time on one of your next grocery store visits to evaluate the products you usually buy against other identical products and create a new set of healthier staples. If you are buying bread for example, compare the bread you usually buy to an equivalent bread that may have better nutritional factors. Does one have less fat? Fewer sugars? Higher protein content? Once you identify healthier items, take this opportunity to adjust your purchases for the future.

Everything you purchase that comes in a box, can or plastic wrap should be evaluated. Don't confuse the butcher department, however, with the deli. Packaged luncheon meats and processed cheese foods should be avoided whenever possible. In most instances, these items contain high quantities of sodium, fat, cancer-causing nitrites and preservatives.

Our goal is to make you think about what you eat and question anything that does not appear to be logical. If you don't do it already, start reading the labels for all the packaged products you buy. When you do not read labels, you can unknowingly be eating things that you should really avoid. By law, manufacturers are supposed to disclose all of the ingredients that are in their foods prominently on the "supplement panel". Unfortunately, manufacturers do NOT need to list any chemical reactions those ingredients may have when various ingredients are mixed together. In other words, you know that hydrogen and nitrogen, when mixed together, will create a bomb. But, if that bomb were a food, it would be legal for a manufacturer to list both hydrogen and nitrogen as ingredients, yet they would not be required to disclose that consuming the two together will cause you to explode!

A perfect example of this deception is deep-fried items or items cooked at very high temperatures like pizza. When foods are deep fried or baked extra hot, cancer-causing acrylamide is released in the process. Acrylamide content does not need to be disclosed to you on the label because acrylamide was not an ingredient that was added to the product by the manufacturer. It was simply a result of the process in which the product was produced, thereby not requiring disclosure to you.

Other terms that mean something different than you would assume are things like "natural". Although a manufacturer can only say "100% natural" if the item has no artificial ingredients, the term "natural flavoring" does not mean the flavors you are tasting are of natural origin. It means that chemicals have been strategically mixed to create the natural flavor you would expect to taste for that item. I know it sounds confusing, but that's how it works. Let me give you an example using low-grade hamburger. Most low-grade hamburger meat has very little flavor of its own or it has an unsavory, undesirable one. That is why chemical flavor enhancers are used in order for your burger to taste more like better quality beef. This same kind of flavor enhancement can be used for any item. Fruit drinks, chocolate treats, and much of the packaged foods you may be eating have been made to taste the way they do by adding "natural flavoring" that is anything but "natural".

"Organic" is another term that is being used to trick the consumer into thinking an item is healthy. From the government's legal perspective, the term "organic" on a label simply means that a product's ingredients are at least 95% free of pesticides, hormones, irradiation and bioengineering. However, it does NOT mean that it is healthy, free of added chemicals or is good for you. Because the consumer attaches the word "organic" with "healthy", manufacturers are now capitalizing on our naiveté and wantonly using the term to motivate our purchase of otherwise unhealthy junk foods. The "organic" term originated to help us differentiate between commercially grown fruits, vegetables, chicken or meat products and those that were grown without pesticides, hormones, irradiation or bioengineering.

Historically we have been willing to pay more for organic produce, chicken or organic beef because we recognize that it costs more to produce these items naturally. But, these same considerations don't even apply to manufactured concoctions such as Oreo cookie copies, high sugar cereals and even frozen chocolate waffles. Even so, companies that make these sugary snack and junk food items now boast soaring sales since the term "organic" was placed on their labels even though the nutritional content is no better than their "non-organic" counterpart. Instead of being a means for consumer protection and wise purchasing, the term "organic" is now being used as a commercial sales tool. And, in most instances, we are paying more for the privilege of purchasing these new "organic" foods even though there is generally no additional expense to their manufacture.

"Low fat," "lite" and "lean" are all terms that can be misleading. Rather than depend upon the manufacturer's promotional lingo prominently displayed on the front of a package to tell you if their product is healthy, simply read the nutritional information provided on the "supplemental facts" panel. Keep one thing in mind; the main thing that concerns you is the fat-to-calorie ratio and the content of chemical ingredients in the product. However, you should also be aware if the product is high in sugar and carbohydrates or if there is any protein value.

Ideally, your daily fat consumption should not exceed 30% of your total calorie count each day. When you look at the supplement panel on each of the foods you buy, it will tell you the number of calories per serving. It will then tell you the number of fat calories per serving. Be sure that the fat calories do not exceed 30% of the total calories for that item. For example, if you pick wheat crackers and it shows "25 calories per serving" and "7 fat calories per serving", one serving of crackers would be 28% fat which is under 30% fat making it acceptable to eat. If you are eating fresh fruits and vegetables, or fresh meats from the butcher department, you need not worry about their fat content. Generally speaking, nature provides for your health by not exceeding the 30% rule.

When you shop at the grocery store, you can avoid most of the processed foods and unhealthy fare just by shopping around the perimeter of your market and eliminating the aisles. Most markets are set up the same way. The produce section includes fresh fruits and vegetables. This moves into the dairy section which includes milk, eggs, cheese and deli items. Then comes the fresh butcher's department with meats, poultry and fish followed by the baked goods section full of breads, rolls and pastry.

Obviously, it takes a lot of willpower and a certain amount of practicality to avoid the aisles. Cleaning supplies and paper goods alone will force you to venture down those rows. If you find yourself in a food aisle, be smart in your purchases. Avoid items containing a lot of chemicals. You will easily identify those products by the long list of ingredients that you cannot pronounce. You also want to stay away from items containing a lot of sodium, saturated and hydrogenated fats. When you read the labels, you can easily find low fat, healthy options to fill your grocery cart.

Be label wise. Know what you are putting into your body. The basic rule when evaluating any of the ingredients in something you consider eating: If you cannot pronounce it... Don't Eat It!

## GOOD FATS AND BAD

Fats are easy and somewhat obvious to address.  Everyone is pretty much aware that low fat diets are healthier than high fat ones.  But, there's a lot more to it than that. Although much attention has been focused on the need to reduce dietary fat, the body requires moderate amounts of it. During infancy and childhood, fat is necessary for normal brain development. Throughout life, fat is essential to provide energy and support physical growth. However, after about two years of age, the body requires only small amounts of fat - generally less than is consumed in the average diet.

Fat is an essential nutrient that plays several vital roles.  It:

- Regenerates skin, nails and body oils
- Regulates the body by forming hormones
- Insulates and pads internal organs
- Carries fat-soluble vitamins throughout the body
- Helps repair damaged tissue
- Fights infections
- Is an energy source

Fats are the way the body stores energy.  When storage areas like overweight hips, thighs or stomach are overloaded,  the body slows down and loses power. Excessive fat intake is a major contributor to health disorders such as overweight, high blood pressure, coronary heart disease and colon cancer.

To understand how fat intake is related to health problems, it is necessary to understand the different types of fats available and the ways in which these fats act within the body.  Natural fats are composed of building blocks called "fatty acids".

There are three major categories of fatty acids:

* Saturated          * Polyunsaturated        * Monounsaturated

These classifications are based on the number of hydrogen atoms in the chemical structure of a given molecule of fatty acid. Some fats are good. Some are not.

**SATURATED FATS** are found primarily in animal products, including dairy items. Whole milk, cream and cheese in addition to meats like beef, veal, lamb, pork, and ham all contain saturated fats. Some vegetable products, including coconut oil, palm kernel oil, and vegetable shortening are also high in saturated fat.

Saturated fats enhance the manufacture of cholesterol by the liver. Therefore, excessive dietary intake of saturated fats can significantly raise your blood cholesterol level, especially the level of low-density lipoproteins (LDL's) or "bad cholesterol". Your daily intake of saturated fats should be kept below 10% of your total calorie intake daily. However, for people who have severe problems with high-blood cholesterol, even that level may be too high.

**POLYUNSATURATED FATS** are primarily found in corn, soybean, safflower and sunflower oils. Certain fish oils are also high in polyunsaturates. Unlike the saturated fats, polyunsaturates may actually lower total blood cholesterol levels. In doing so, however, large amounts of polyunsaturates also have a tendency to reduce high density lipoproteins (HDL's) which is the "good cholesterol" your body needs.

**MONOUNSATURATED FATS** are found mostly in vegetables and nut oils such as olives and peanuts. These fats appear to reduce blood levels of LDL's (bad) without affecting HDL's (good) in any way, although the positive impact upon LDL cholesterol is relatively modest.

# WATCH OUT FOR MANUFACTURED FATS

**TRANS FATS** are produced when food manufacturers take liquid vegetable oils, heat them and add metal catalysts and hydrogen to the mix in order to solidify it as an oil so it can be made to resemble real food such as butter. This process is called "hydrogenation". It produces hardened vegetable oils that remain solid at room temperature and are made into shortening and margarine. The purpose behind this process is purely monetary for food manufacturers and has no health benefit. It is actually quite harmful. In fact, hydrogenation actually ruins the nutritional value of vegetable oils. Because the chemical composition of these fats are shaped differently from natural fatty acids, the body doesn't recognize what to do with them and they eventually block arteries and other organ function.

Over the last 50 years, trans fats have become one of the most common ingredients in both grocery store and restaurant fare because it enables foods to stay fresh longer, oftentimes without expensive refrigeration requirements. The Food & Drug Administration is alarmed that Americans are unaware of the dangers of trans fats and product labels do not identify them as such. They estimate that simple labeling could save at least $1 billion dollars in annual healthcare costs by preventing 6,400 cases of heart disease per year and at least 2,100 deaths. Other studies have shown that trans fatty acids are responsible for about 30,000 premature deaths per year.

## *You Can Avoid Over-Eating Trans Fat*

Unfortunately, not all food labels break out its fat content. By law, all labels will list grams of fat, but will not necessarily tell you WHAT KIND of fat can be found in that food item. It is also important to note that hidden trans fats are generally not included in the label's fat totals for most products. Highly processed foods have a much more likely chance of containing unwanted fats than natural food items bought in the fresh butcher department or produce section of your grocery store.

The average American eats about 34 grams a day of saturated and trans fats combined. This is well over the recommended daily intake of 20 grams of saturated fat for an average 2000 calorie-per-day diet. It is almost impossible to calculate the actual amount of trans fats present in the foods we eat since they are not listed on the supplement panel of most packaged food and will not be mandated unless legislation is passed requiring disclosure.

The best way to avoid eating trans fats is to avoid processed foods or foods containing shortening whenever possible. That would include items such as:

* margarine          * crackers
* cheese food (Velveeta)   * cookies
* fish sticks         * French fries
* cereals            * chips
* cakes             * muffins

The fast food industry has been under scrutiny about the health hazard their food presents to the public. Undisclosed fats used to extend food shelf life have been the cause of many law suits and it is predicted that the fast food industry will soon become another tobacco industry fiasco when it comes to class action suits. It is one thing when a consumer makes an adult decision to use a product that will knowingly compromise their health. It is another when we are teaching our children that they will find "comfort, friends and family" when they frequent fast food restaurants. These places are promoted as the "Happy place to be", but, they are not letting the public know that their establishment may be seriously detrimental to everyone's health at the same time.

Become more aware of the marketing used to promote convenient, snack & junk food items. Almost without exception, marketing is targeted at children and plays on a parent's guilt over time restrictions and obligations that take them away from parenting availability. The promise of good times, good friends, happy feelings and warm memories are all incorporated into each very expensive promotional ad campaign. Billions of dollars are spent each year promoting products that are clearly threatening to our health, yet we never seem to question their message or their motive. Even though we may feel skepticism and distrust over the big pharmaceutical company's true concern for the public's health, we do not seem to extend the same distrust to big food companies like Kraft or General Foods. Do you really think these giant food conglomerates care about your health when they are responsible for filling their products with hidden fats that can ultimately kill consumers?

# ESSENTIAL FATTY ACIDS MAKE A HEALTHY SUPPLEMENT

Essential Fatty Acids (also known as EFA's) are critical to health, physical devel-opment and weight loss. They are the "good fats" needed to lubricate the body's organs, provide structural use, act as hormonal couriers and enhance skin, hair and nail quality. Since the body does not produce its own essential fatty acids, they must be obtained through diet. When absent or deficient, the body will store unwanted body fat in its place, making weight loss and good health more diffi-cult. In addition, proper EFA consumption increases metabolic rate and fat burn-ing ability to better facilitate weight loss.

Essential fatty acids are broken down primarily into omega-6 and omega-3's. Omega-6's are easily available in commonly eaten foods such as corn, safflower, soy, sunflower, oils made from these items, as well as margarine, almost all baked goods, plus most fried fast food and "junk" foods. Omega-3 fatty acids, howev-er, are found in more limited sources like fish, flax, walnuts, Brazil nuts, and dried beans. Obtaining this important nutrient is difficult in adequate quantities making daily supplementation very important.

There are three major contributions that omega-3 fatty acids make specifically for weight loss. They increase metabolic rate, therefore burning more fat and glu-cose; provide the "good fats" the body needs which makes stored body fat avail-able for elimination as well as increasing good hormones which help the kidneys to eliminate excess salt and water.

Essential fatty acids are particularly effective for people on any kind of hormone therapy, for arthritis sufferers or any person who tends to store excess fat due to chemical complications associated with prescription medications. In addition to weight loss affects, it is essential that you take EFA's daily because they are part of every cell membrane in the body and are needed for healthy cell repair. EFA's are also critical for brain development, health of the nervous system (the brain is 60-70% fat), are a source of energy and are pre-cursors to most adrenal gland, sex hormones and numerous inter-cellular messenger molecules.

Fats are important for body balance and all fats are not bad. They are essential to good health. But, the key is the type of fat you consume. The popular concept in traditional dieting that assumes "fat makes you fat" is simply not true. Over the past thirty years, America has been on low-fat diet programs but are more obese today than ever before. Low-fat and no-fat diets have only contributed to more obesity in our country. People are substituting carbohydrates and sugar in place of fat but, carbohydrates and sugar are what activates hormones to store fat.

Indirectly, much of the success people experienced on the original Atkin's Diet was due to elevated essential fatty acid consumption associated with the high fat allowance his program provided. Unlimited dairy, heavy cream, bacon and salami are not healthy but collectively boosted essential fatty acid levels which, in turn, boosted weight loss. Unfortunately, regular consumption of high fat foods such as these also provide an imbalance of omega 6 to omega 3 fatty acids which raises cholesterol levels and creates a toxic load on the liver and kidneys. This is just another reason why people have a hard time sustaining Atkin's eating guidelines.

You should also be aware that omega-3 essential fatty acid deficiencies are also associated with acne, hair loss, dry, bumpy skin, dry, brittle hair, hormonal problems, impaired growth and poor immune function. All of these could result in chronic infections or cancer, poor wound healing, fertility problems, mental challenges, depression, and kidney dysfunction.

## Why Do EFA's Work?
Essential fatty acids become part of your cell membranes and positively affect the way your cells behave. Consequently, the health of your cells will have a direct reflection on the health of your body. EFA's improve your cell's response to insulin, neurotransmitters and other messengers. They are essential for the repair process when cells are damaged and they provide the 'good fats' your body needs to lubricate your organs and promote overall cellular health.

Americans consume a dangerously low amount of omega 3's. Essential fatty acids are minimally available in most foods and that is why supplementation becomes critical. Omega 3 fatty acids come from fish and marine oils. They contain two important varieties: "EPA" (eicosapentaenoic acid), and "DHA" (decosahexaenoic acid). Both varieties are critical for a number of reasons. But, because people do not generally eat adequate quantities of the foods containing omega 3 fatty acids (seafood), supplements are needed.

## Why Is Flaxseed Oil Not As Affective As EFA'S?
"EPA" has the greatest benefits in reducing the risk of heart disease and "DHA" affects vision, brain, and nerve function. Flaxseed oil does not contain "EPA" or "DHA". It is rich in alpha-linolenic acid and, although similar in structure, the

benefits of alpha-linolenic acid are not the same nor are they as effective. Studies have shown that fish oils (EFA's) are much more effective in cellular development and heart health than the acid in flaxseed oil.

Alpha-linolenic acid converts rapidly into "EPA" in the body, and more slowly into "DHA". Unfortunately, other fats consumed in processed foods, like trans-fats, can stop the conversion of these necessary fatty acids leaving you unprotected. That is why it is important that you take an essential fatty acid supplement that already contains the necessary "EPA" and "DHA" needed, and doesn't require any conversion in order for your body to obtain a proper supply.

### Are All Essential Fatty Acids The Same?
No. Fatty acids come from marine oils (fish) and are subject to the metal contaminates found in the seafood environment. Be sure the EFA product you select comes from a company that screens for mercury and heavy metal contamination. This is an expensive process that is overlooked by many over-the-counter supplement products.

### Do I Need Omega 6 Fatty Acids?
No, not in supplementation form. The foods you eat contain adequate amounts of omega 6's. It is important to keep omega 6 fatty acid intake low, as it can be counterproductive to many of the benefits of omega 3's. The best way to minimize omega 6 fatty acids in your diet is to avoid all vegetable seed oils and those products that contain them.

# The Country Club Diet

## Preparing For Change & Staying Motivated

# THE COUNTRY CLUB DIET

*The Country Club Diet* is not about willpower. It is about empowering you with the right information so that you can make informed and healthy decisions about your life and the way you eat. You are not weak. There is nothing wrong with you. You do not have a character flaw that causes you to have health problems or to be overweight. Your body is normal and it is reacting normally to the imbalanced food and media bombardment that leaves everyone in a state of confusion while misdirecting their food choices. This program is about empowerment and knowledge. When you know the right things to do in order to look good, feel strong and get healthy, it will be a lot easier for you to make the right choices.

Most likely you have been unaware before now of the impact the food you eat has on your body. Like most Americans, you have probably failed at numerous attempts to achieve weight loss goals in the past. By learning the value of each required change necessary to obtain the healthy body you desire, you can learn to prefer new behaviors over old ones. You should not feel any feelings of blame or guilt over your historical actions. You now have the ability to create a game plan for your success.

You are responsible for your body's health. This book will help you to create your own personal plan for changes that is both sensible, workable and fits within your own personal lifestyle. Both science and technology are behind the results achieved with *The Country Club Die*t because it treats the entire body, both mentally and physically, in order to create maximum balance.

### THINK CHANGE...
**"You can't solve a problem with the same mind that created it."**
**Thomas Edison**

Developing emotional willingness and preparation are key to the success of anyone desirous of making healthy changes. People who try to accomplish changes they are not prepared to make set themselves up for eventual failure. The beauty of this program is that it allows the reader to customize it for themselves. No two people are exactly the same. Your willingness and readiness for change will establish how rapidly or slowly you will proceed toward your individual goal. Dietary changes are a very small facet of this program. Our approach takes into account your genetics, activity level, hormone balance, medical history, environmental influences, toxins, blood, bowel and liver function, infections, plus emotional and psychological stressors.

Change happens slowly, but it is possible for you to regain control over your life and your health. New habits, like old ones, are established over time. For you to become successful long-term, your new habits must become preferred to your old. They must become part of your automatic and unconscious behavioral response system.

This book will provide you with a specific set of guidelines that can assist you throughout your self-changing journey. We have now put into practical practice, techniques that experts have identified as early as 1983 to change behavior in order to facilitate weight loss and create a healthier and more fit body. We feel it is time to address this critical issue from its true psychological source rather than simply treat the physical 'condition' of being overweight. Poor health and increased weight is a result of long-established eating and behavioral patterns. Good health and weight loss is a result of healthy nutrition and exercise.

In order for a program to be successful long-term, it must address five key factors; stabilize sugar and insulin in your body, activate your metabolism, control appetite, promote exercise and help you become mentally prepared for change without stress. Most commercial weight loss plans only address one or two of these factors. They typically treat the 'symptoms' of an overweight condition and not the cause. Every person is a biochemically different and solitary individual. They have different issues and unique combinations of stressors that cause his or her health problems. To achieve your desired fat loss result, mental preparation is essential along with total chemical body balance that can best be created through proper diet, exercise and nutritional supplements. Most diets work in the short-term. But, to achieve permanent, long-term weight management success, realistic dietary and lifestyle changes must be made.

## *Discourage Your Desire To Proceed Quickly*

Personal challenges, family or emotional issues, fear, or any number of other factors may cause you to slow down your progress. There is no time-line for this process. The beauty of *The Country Club Diet* is that it works at YOUR pace.

Most people lose weight or make dietary changes for one of two reasons: vanity or fear. They are either unhappy with the way they look or their doctor has presented concerns for their physical health, or both. It is important that you understand that your personal motivation DOES NOT mean that you are ready for action. It is not unusual for you to be so concerned about your potential health complications or are desirous of looking better as quickly as possible that you become over-zealous in your enthusiasm. At this time, be aware of how you feel and be easy on yourself. The more your changes come from inside you and not from external sources, the more effective and successful they will be.

Unless you are both mentally and physically prepared for your weight loss and wellness experience, you will fail quickly and become defeated in the process. Take this time to educate yourself about the benefits for each of the specific changes you will need to make. Too many changes at one time will quickly become overwhelming and unmanageable. This may be a time when you will need to slow down your tendency for action and minimize changes to diet & exercise schedules. Success comes in the achievement, not in the time in which it takes to make it happen.

Most people are very motivated when they initially decide to address their weight issues. However, making too many changes all at one time will be neither manageable nor effective. Empowerment comes with success and ease. Little changes are much easier to fit into one's lifestyle than dramatic ones. Even though you will be planning many changes along the way, please do not allow yourself to implement those changes until you feel you are completely ready.

# CREATING AN ACTION PLAN

Identify your challenges and find workable solutions for each one. Write them down. Be very specific for each entry. If you have a problem food, for example, you can identify replacement options then decide what is the most desirable replacement item for you. Make a plan for every problem area that you may have that includes stress triggers, food choices, exercise, etcetera. Every aspect of your lifestyle, as it relates to your eating, needs to be reviewed thoroughly. Start from the time you get up in the morning until you go to bed. Do not feel that you must create this plan in one day. This will be created after a lot of time, personal reflection and contemplation takes place. Please remember, you will not be implementing all of the alternative behaviors you are constructing in the planning phase all at one time. While planning, the thought of all of these changes may feel overwhelming. But, don't allow that to happen. You are making progress even in your evaluation. You can implement your changes one day at a time.

Once your Action Plan is finalized, be sure to put a copy at each location that may be appropriate. The kitchen, your bedroom, even your office should have a copy of your plan for easy reference. You created the plan. You need to keep it handy so you can remind yourself of the alternative actions you have set for the various circumstances that may arise. Your plan will also serve as a reminder of your commitment to take responsibility for carrying out the plan you have created.

Simply deciding to do something positive in order to lose weight and improve your health is an accomplishment all by itself. Recognizing this first step is a giant leap toward your health goal.

To begin, start with your weight history. What programs have you been on before? Identify what needs to happen in order for you to feel you can be successful with this program now. List the criteria that needs to be in place. Some of them may be:

- ✔ Simplicity - easy to follow
- ✔ Allows you to dine out
- ✔ Must include dessert
- ✔ Needs to understand why each change is beneficial
- ✔ Needs support - my family doesn't support me
- ✔ Must find support from an outside source

Your list of the specific criteria that needs to be in place in order for you to be successful at achieving your goal will enable you to avoid the pitfalls you have experienced from previous programs. Learning from your mistakes makes each new attempt at success a little easier.

Identify Your Eating Habits. Once you have identified patterns in the way you eat, specifically indicate what alterations may need to be made in order to break those patterns that are counter-productive to your goal. How will you make them? What actions or foods will replace bad behaviors or poor dietary choices?

What kind of eater are you?: Good? Bad? Healthy? Fast Food? Snacker?

What is your overall Goal? Do you want to:

- Eat small, healthier portions more often?
- Avoid snacking?
- Identify the best times of the day to eat? ✓
- Find healthy snacks to fill the void between meals? ✓

## KNOW YOUR REASONS WHY

Understanding any challenge you are faced with is key to solving it. If you do not acknowledge the cause of your problems, how can you come up with a resolution to solve them? By being clear about your history, you have taken a giant step toward ensuring that you will not self-sabotage your current self-improvement efforts.

a. Why are you overweight? _____

_____
_____
_____
_____

b. Why is achieving your goal important to you? _____

_____
_____
_____

c. Why are you concerned about your current health condition?

_____
_____
_____
_____
_____

d. Why are you concerned about how other people see you?

_____
_____
_____
_____
_____
_____

# CREATING COMMITMENT

Once your evaluation is complete and the basic plan for change has been established, you still have a little homework to do before putting your plan into action. Commitment includes not only a willingness to act, but also developing your belief in your ability to change. This comfort level for achievement should be reinforced every day. When your belief in your ability begins to falter, you must immediately step back and shore-up all the successful changes made up until that time.

**Identify Benefits**: If there are any serious behavior or nutritional changes that are difficult for you to make, create a list of all the benefits associated with making that specific change. This will enable you to refer to 'why' you want to eat certain things, act a certain way or exercise when you have not been previously motivated to do so.

**Make Change A Priority:** As you go through and review your plan for change, identify a date when you think changes for specific items should be implemented. Once made, those changes need to be maintained. Be sure that you do not assign more than three changes on any given date, nor do you place the next date for change within ten days of the first. Depending upon the severity of the changes, you may even have months between the first and the next adjustment. This is **your** plan. It needs to be implemented at your pace.

**Tell Everyone:** Tell friends and family of your intention and commitment to a 'healthier' and 'lighter' lifestyle. Confirm everyone's support and belief in the goals you have set. Be sure to communicate the kind of support you are looking for from friends and family. People who care about you can only help when they know how. Tell them exactly what you would like for them to do, such as…

> ✔ Don't keep asking how I am doing.
> ✔ Don't nag me.
> ✔ Don't condemn me when I mess up.
> ✔ Offer to help when I look overwhelmed.
> ✔ Tell me you're proud of me for doing this.

**Be Aware That Outside Influences Affect You Too.** It is not unusual for family members or friends to take your weight loss efforts for granted. This is especially true when you have tried multiple programs or various 'diets' over a long period of time. In order to keep these people on your team, you need to let them know where they fit into your plan. Like any good game, you need an objective, goal, rules for direction and support.

**Where Did You Go Wrong Before?** Be aware of the pitfalls associated with previous weight loss attempts and be sure to address those in order to avoid the same results this time. When you control your hunger and elevate your metabolism by getting your hormones in balance and eat in a healthy and sensible manner, weight loss can be fast and easy. Do not beat yourself up mentally because you have not been successful losing weight in the past. You're doing everything right this time. Unwanted pounds and inches will simply disappear.

# EMOTIONAL EATING & OVERCOMING STRESS

For many, stress, even 'good stress', can cause nervous eating. When you find yourself frustrated or angry and headed for the kitchen, first ask the following questions:

◄ **Does food take away my frustrations?**
◄ **How will I feel if I don't eat items that I don't need?**
◄ **What can I do instead of eat?**

**You Must Start To:**

**Deal With Stress & Anxiety:** The more confident you are about the changes you are going to make, the less anxiety you will feel. Anxiety and stress are real. They can only be conquered when they are understood and countered with realistic options. Proper diet and exercise will go a long way to assist you with stress management.

**Work With Real Feelings.** Rather than say "I feel fat", take out the word "fat" because it is not an emotion, it is a physical state. Identify what EMOTION is bothering you so you can deal directly with that.

**Make A "To Do" List.** Keeping busy and well organized can eliminate a lot of stress. As you begin to see progress while checking off the items on your list, the various tasks you have designed for yourself will not seem so overwhelming and you can achieve a wonderful sense of accomplishment in the process.

**Take A 10-minute Time Out.** Wait 10 minutes before turning to food in times of stress. You can then use that 10 minutes to determine who or what is the appropriate target of your frustrations and find a solution that satisfies you without using food as an escape. If you turn to food too quickly, you'll only be angry at yourself later.

**Call A Friend.** Just talking-out anger or frustrations to a caring ear will make you feel better and eliminate any potential feelings of isolation and of being alone.

**Eliminate Other People's Expectations.** Everyone must live for themselves. Construct positive walls against negative energies from others. Be sure to set your own goals and not the goals of family and friends.

**Make Pleasure A Priority.** Take up an activity that has no practical application. Sculpture, sewing, jewelry making, bird watching, park sitting, are all options. When stressed, turn toward your hobby instead of food. You need to plan your activities with YOU in mind, not anyone else. Learn to be responsible for yourself and the achievement of your dreams. If a well-meaning friend dumps water on your vision to lose weight, try to be understanding and say nothing. A heckler often has their own ax to grind and may be jealous of your success.

**Think Positive Thoughts.** Negative thoughts can have the same visualization power as positive ones. When you think negative thoughts about yourself such as, "I have no willpower", that can become a self-fulfilling prophecy. Don't let this happen to you. Look at the good in everything you do. Don't be angry at yourself for splurging a little. Recognize that you ate less of that item than you would have in the past.

**Staying Motivated** is a big part of your health and weight loss effort... especially if you have a substantial amount of weight to lose. People will treat you in the manner in which you demand to be treated. For most of us, we have been lax in making our demands known. This is your time to shine. You have a vision, a plan and a goal for yourself. You have made a commitment to make changes for the better in your life. Do not let anyone stand in the way of achieving your goals. You have the power to achieve your dreams... USE IT!

# TAKE ACTION

Although you are mentally prepared, change is still implemented slowly. Known dietary challenges are once again reviewed and adjustments are introduced incrementally. Too many changes at one time can be overwhelming even though you think you are ready to take action. If you have not been exercising, for example, it needs to be introduced slowly. Don't attempt a daily workout at the onset. Exercising one or two days a week for a short duration of time would be the initial action prescribed. As you become comfortable and in control of your workout day or other changes you have implemented, then additional changes can be introduced.

Even when you have done all the necessary preparation, there are no guarantees that each of your planned actions will be successful. Being aware of the pitfalls that may arise will greatly increase your chance of success. Every day will not be easy. Some changes will be more painful or more difficult than others. Every troubled or problematic behavior must have a healthy substitute that you can embrace and live with or you will return to old patterns.

**Follow Your Time-Line.** You have created specific dates when behaviors should be altered. Try to stay on that calendar. You have made an emotional commitment to that plan and you do not want to make a lot of adjustments, if possible. If you are progressing well, do not be too anxious to move ahead too quickly.

**Active Diversions.** Diversions should be a big part of the action phase. Select preferred diversions for negative behaviors. New challenges will always arise as plans are put into action. Diversions for inappropriate eating or snacking may be reading, cleaning, playing piano, creating a hobby. You can cook, knit or sew, have sex, exercise, walk or simply call a friend. Your options are endless.

**Relaxation.** Relaxing should be part of your action plan. Watching television is NOT considered relaxation. Meditation, prayer, yoga and progressive muscle relaxation are best and should be conducted in a quiet environment. Get into a comfortable position, focus on yourself internally and let go of all anxieties. Just ten to twenty minutes of quiet meditation will provide you with increased energy, increased alpha (pleasurable) brain waves, decreased blood pressure & muscle tension, decreased stress, improved sleep, improved concentration and improved health. WOW!

**Counter-Thinking.** Be aware of your view of yourself. Irrational self-statements can undermine the best of intentions. It promotes negative thoughts which result in negative behaviors. Counter-thinking can also provide a dose of reality to otherwise irrational assumptions. For example:

| YOUR THOUGHT... | COUNTER THOUGHT... |
|---|---|
| I can't control my eating. | I don't have to let my eating control me. |
| I need to eat to make me feel better. | A short, quiet walk would do me good now. |
| I should be competent in everything. | There is so much I still have to learn |
| Why do I always have to fail? | Look how far I've come. |
| I've only lost 12 pounds. | I am 12 pounds lighter! |
| I hate making changes. | These changes are so much better for me. |

Do not allow yourself to confuse DESIRES for NEEDS. You may "want" to eat a pizza. But, you really "need" to eat protein like chicken.

**Promote Your Own Value.** You are WORTH all of the effort you are putting into your program. You have value. Many people who suffer from overweight conditions begin to question their worth which can be very defeating. Recognize your ongoing accomplishments without pressuring yourself to do more. You need to be making change for yourself... not for family or friends. If you are making changes for someone else and you have a bad day, you now run the risk of letting down someone you care about and you never want to feel that way. Life isn't perfect. There will be good days and bad. But, no matter what, you need to recognize that you are important and that your accomplishments count. You have been successful just by virtue of the fact that you are making a commitment to make a difference in your own life.

# ELIMINATE TEMPTATION

The best way to fight behaviors you are trying to change is to eliminate the temptations that precipitate those behaviors whenever possible. You know what triggers drive you to the refrigerator. If it's too hard to avoid the automatic response stress or upset causes, then at least be sure that your usual array of tempting treats are unavailable.

- ◄ Do not keep high calorie/high fat foods in the house.
- ◄ Do not purchase or stock white starches.
- ◄ Only eat desserts when dining out.
- ◄ Stock frozen yogurt instead of ice cream.
- ◄ Keep healthy snack options on hand.

You cannot eat what is unavailable to you. Pantries and refrigerators should be cleaned out and all inappropriate snacks and food items removed. This is also the perfect time to check expiration dates for oils, dressings, spices and other condiments.

### Responsibly Reward Changed Behavior

Identify non-food rewards for positive behaviors. Reinforcement for good changes needs to be part of your program. You do not want to punish yourself for properly resisting temptation. It will weaken your resistance and increase your risk of relapse. Reward yourself. Do something special every week to help you celebrate that week's successes. A reward can be something as little as a relaxing afternoon in the sun. Go get a massage or dine out at a special place. You can even create an affordable 'payment' to yourself each week for good behavior and place it in a 'good behavior shopping account' for a future spending spree! After all, it won't be long and you'll need smaller clothes!

### Update Your Action Plan

It is important that you make a written commitment to your changes in the form of your action plan. This plan may be altered depending upon you're your ability to comply with the items you thought would be workable when your plan was created. When changes to your plan are made, be sure you not only identify the alternative behavior, you must also identify the behavior you wish to change. For example:

| BAD BEHAVIOR | NEW ALTERNATIVE BEHAVIOR |
|---|---|
| Eat ice cream | Eat low-fat frozen yogurt |
| Snack when stressed | Take a short walk, read, call a friend |
| Love white bread | Buy only whole wheat & rye |

As a reminder, you can also keep a sign on the face of your refrigerator that lists your new alternative behaviors so you can be immediately re-directed prior to taking an action you may regret later. So many times we do things out of habit. If new, preferred behaviors are not in the forefront of your mind, old patterns will quickly reappear.

# EVALUATE YOUR SUCCESS

This is the most important part of your process, evaluating your success. Every pound, every inch, every dietary change that benefits your body, every environmental change that uplifts your spirit, even taking your vitamins every day, all contribute to your overall effort of regaining balance and harmony in your body and your life. Do not take these changes lightly, no matter how small they appear. Collectively, they will make a monumental difference in the quality of your life and your ability to see for yourself, how powerful and successful a person you really are:

a. How much smaller are you getting? _____

    _____

b. What permanent dietary changes have you made?

    _____

    _____

c. How much 'junk food' have you cut from your diet?

    _____

    _____

d.  How do you feel physically? _____
_____
_____

e.  Do you feel you have more energy?
_____
_____

f.  Are you exercising regularly? _____
_____

g.  Are people beginning to notice a difference in your appearance?
_____
_____

h.  Are you happy with your progress? _____
_____
_____

i.  What do you need to do next to make your program more successful?
_____
_____
_____

# SUCCESS TIPS

As a recap, here are the key elements that will provide you with better health, a leaner body and a brighter tomorrow:

◀  Eat frequent, smaller meals.

◀  Focus on high protein / low starchy carbohydrate meal plans.

◀  Take daily nutritional supplements as needed.

◀  Exercise.

◀  Find a buddy for exercise and/or weight loss efforts.

◀  Keep unwanted foods out of refrigerator & pantry.

◀  Read labels and shop smart.

◀  Rearrange your home.  Make it less stressful.  Create quiet areas.

◀  Keep a diary.  Write down goals as well as progress made.

◀  Look for complements.

◀  Encourage friends & family members to encourage you.

◀  Communicate.  What help do you need?  How can others help you?

◀  Minimize guilt.

◀  Listen to your body.

◀  Analyze how you feel.

◀  Stay positive.

# TRADING POUNDS

We live in a world desirous of immediate gratification. Anytime we make changes, no matter what the change, we want to see immediate results. That's why painting a room is so satisfactory. Ten minutes after you start, you can already see an improvement. And, an hour or two later... voila!

Weight loss isn't a race. You need to stop and recognize that each pound you lose is another segment of your newly painted wall. Unfortunately, every pound lost will not necessarily show on the scale. Friends and family may not be an indicator either. Not everyone around you sees that your pants are now looser or that you have tightened your belt another notch. But YOU do, and that's what's important.

Since you are restructuring your meals and are making protein the mainstay of your diet, it will not be unusual for you to see a reduction in inches without a pound change on the scale. Fat loss is your goal. After a few weeks you will be losing fat, but may be 'trading pounds'.

The impact of a protein increase in your diet means the rebuilding of muscle mass that has been lost while on other diet programs. Lean muscle mass weighs five times more than fat for the same physical size. When your body becomes leaner, it actually becomes heavier even though your body fat percentage is greatly reduced. We have worked with people who have reported that they have gone from a high of 37% body fat to as low as 17% and are HEAVIER, but trimmer than they were when previously at the same goal weight. It is also common for people to see a drastic reduction in inches indicated by clothing sizes with a minimum of pounds lost.

Trading pounds means that you are replacing fat with lean muscle. Eating more protein and exercising to maximize fat burn will greatly affect your body fat percentage. To best identify your true progress, measure your waist & hips and keep a record of the inches lost. Pay attention to how your clothes fit. A drop in pant size is much more valid than a declining scale.

# SUSTAINING YOUR LOSS

This is the most critical phase for long-term success. Constant reinforcement of improved behaviors is required here. Your potential to slip back into old behaviors is high once you reach your weight goal. You may be over-confident in your ability to succeed. Sabotaging your success in the form of 'rewards' like, "I deserve some of my old favorite treats," can cause you to unintentionally slip back into old habits. The reward systems established while you are losing unwanted fat should be reinforced and continued in practice after you reach your target weight. Achieving your weight loss goal does not mean that old food and behavior practices can be reestablished. Eating right is not a "temporary diet", it is a lifestyle that needs to be continued in order for your new lean and healthy body to be maintained.

Relapse of some sort is inevitable. Minimize the guilt associated with the occasional relapse and get back on track as quickly as possible. Maintaining all the new dietary, lifestyle and exercise behaviors that were put into practice with your Action Plan needs to become your preferred way of life. You will no longer evaluate whether you want to exercise on a particular day, for example, it should become a required behavior if that day is an exercise day.

You should consider yourself on "maintenance" for at least six months from the time your weight loss goal is obtained. The most common threats to maintenance are social pressures, internal challenges and special situations or events that arise. These three factors undermine confidence, conviction and commitment. Since most people have had a history of temporary weight loss, the fear of re-gaining unwanted pounds may sabotage maintenance efforts. Poor eating habits and their associated behaviors generally hold some attraction long after the bad habits are broken. The changed behaviors MUST become your preferred behaviors. It is impossible to remain free of temptations forever. Additionally, supportive family members need to remain supportive and not assume that things will "go back to normal" when your weight loss goal has been achieved.

# RELAPSE TRIGGERS

The three common internal challenges that are closely related to brief lapses in behavior are overconfidence, daily temptations and self-blame.

Lapses in behavior are expected. But, it can be a short ride between a 'lapse' and a 'relapse'. If not closely monitored, a few lapses could push you right back into old behaviors that will cause weight gain and a step backward. Even though you are no longer making changes, maintaining the changes that you have put into action pose their own challenges. Keep your commitment to change strong. Maintaining weight loss is a constant issue for people with weight problems. Personally, I still refer to myself as a "fat person in a thin suit." Many of the emotional triggers that drove me to the refrigerator still occur. But, my new responses to those situations are now different. It's also important to understand that it is much easier for me to respond better now because my body is no longer fighting with my goal. Now that my hormones are healthy, I don't have cravings that could get me into trouble. Even though my 85 pounds has been off more than a decade, I'm still consciously aware that I never want to wear my old "fat suit" ever again.

## *Identify Historical Relapse Patterns*

One of the best ways to fight the inevitability of occasional lapses in behavior is to identify what conditions transpired historically that made you relapse into old patterns and ultimately defeated your weight loss efforts. At this time it is important to recognize the potential for that same condition to exist once again and you want to address it before it causes physical or emotional damage. In this instance, you are in preparation for maintenance. What obstacles do you need to look out for and what is the plan to avoid and / or deal with those obstacles?

Many people will try to give up as soon as they lapse because of the way in which they view the event. When psychological absolutes are put in place and "lapses = failure", it can cause you to becomes guilt ridden with feelings of hopelessness, frustration and stress. These emotions cripple change efforts. With proper preparation, the expectation of the occasional relapse and overcoming it can become an empowering experience and not a negative one.

*Change Is Not Temporary*

Be sure you have not associated some of your changes with temporary actions. Exercise, for example, may be viewed as required behavior in order to lose weight, however, you may think you can discontinue exercising regularly once you reach your weight goal. This is unacceptable. Exercise, healthier foods, revised eating and stress management all play important roles in the maintenance of optimum weight and good health and need to be sustained.

*Maintain The Right Attitude*

Periodically remind yourself of some of your own reasons for wanting to lose weight and be healthy. Use the lists that you have created along the way as reminders. Many of the same motivations will remain in effect along with additional motivations that will be established as your confidence grows. Keeping these factors in the forefront of your mind will allow you to maintain the right attitude about maintaining your changes.

## ESTABLISH A MAINTAINENCE GAME PLAN

**Create a plan to overcome the following challenges:**

1.  What were the major causes of regaining lost weight in the past?
    a.
    b.
    c.

2.  What actions can you plan to take in order to combat historical relapse patterns?
    a.
    b.
    c.

3.  Now that you are more informed about the cycle of change and how it relates to maintaining healthy eating and lifestyle behaviors, what do you think were your biggest challenges to overcome?
    a.
    b.
    c.

4. Do you think you can tolerate a lapse without it turning into a relapse?
   a. Are you emotionally stronger?
   b. Nutritionally healthier?
   c. Confident in your ability to succeed?

5. What do you think you need to do in order to feel more confident?
   a.
   b.
   c.

6. What complications have you prepared yourself for and how will you handle them?
   a.
   b.
   c.

7. Do you have friends or family members that may try to sabotage your success? Who? How can you combat their sabotage efforts?
   a.
   b.
   c.

# Your

# Personal

# Health

## Overcoming

## Deficiencies

# THE DANGERS OF AN OVERWEIGHT CONDITION

Beyond your obvious displeasure with your current weight and health, there are many statistics that show the effects an overweight condition will have on you. For example, according to research conducted by the New York Times, women who gain 10 to 40 pounds after age 35, (an amount considered acceptable under current federal weight guidelines), have an increased risk of suffering a heart attack. A 14-year study conducted by Harvard researchers in 1997 found that weight gains of even 11 to 18 pounds in adult life resulted in a 25% greater chance of suffering or dying of a heart attack. The study evaluated the heart related deaths of more than 115,000 middle aged women and it was concluded that more than 40% of those women experienced heart attacks due to weight gain.

Middle age weight gain is common and deadly. Federal guidelines strongly imply that it is healthy to gain weight as people get older. But, this has many restrictions. When you understand the seriousness of obesity, you are more motivated to make the lifestyle changes necessary to reverse this trend. You owe it to yourself to get in shape.

Every person has an 'ideal body weight' which is derived from a height, weight and bone structure calculation. Your mortality increases as body weight increases or decreases away from your 'ideal weight'. To be blunt, if you deviate from your ideal weight, your chance of ending up dead before your time is greater. Being underweight is actually more hazardous than being overweight because having too little body fat creates even greater stress and risk to the body than being obese.

As a guideline, you can suppose that your life expectancy will be reduced by two to three years for every 10% you are over your 'ideal weight'. Life insurance companies figure on an even higher mortality factor when you are overweight. They calculate that the chance of death is increased by 25% in people who are only 5%-15% over their ideal weight, but is increased by more than 400% in people who are more than 25% over their ideal weight. If you are short, you have an even greater concern because you do not have the same available excess fat distribution as a tall person. Your risk will increase with the ratio of waist to hip measurement so it is critical that you stay as close to your 'ideal weight' as possible.

Although heart problems are most commonly associated with an overweight condition, as we discussed earlier, other life-threatening or life-shortening diseases such as cancer, hypertension, gallbladder disease, lung disorders and diabetes are also high risk possibilities. Breast cancer in women, for example, is 38% more common in patients that are overweight rather than at their ideal weight. And, obesity will push the body into a situation where it is no longer able to control blood sugar levels correctly so that diabetes is developed and daily insulin injections may be required.

Obesity also leaves you susceptible to lower back pain, particularly in men, and may precipitate gout attacks, aggravate arthritic joints, may cause flat feet, contribute to circulatory problems such as varicose veins and respiratory stresses such as shortness of breath and snoring. Hiatus hernias, which usually manifests itself as heartburn, can also become chronic. The diaphragm keeps the esophagus closed except when swallowing, and when the abdominal cavity gets larger because of fat deposits, the diaphragm has some difficulty keeping the tension high enough to stop reverse flow. Antacids will give temporary relief, but losing your extra pounds is a more permanent solution.

Yo-Yo dieting creates an increased health risk because constant weight gain and loss does not enable your body to stabilize and function properly. An overweight condition increases the strain on your heart which is reduced when the excess weight is lost. But, in many cases, some damage to the cardiovascular system will have already occurred. If you continue to gain and lose weight, you may reduce the risk of heart disease when you are closer to your ideal weight, but the ongoing strain and damage to your heart in the process will increase your chance for sudden cardiac death.

If you are a yo-yo dieter, it is our goal to get you to break this trend. The single most important thing you can do when attempting, once again, to reach your ideal weight, is to increase your protein intake rather than reduce your calorie consumption. Standard diets cause you to quickly lose lean tissue from muscle and vital organs which is not replaced during your weight increase stages. That is why you generally feel physically weaker when you diet. Protein is important to fuel your vital organs and rebuild lean muscle mass. In addition, it plays a major role in the brain because it usually contains the precursor amino acids that support and balance the numerous brain messengers such as serotonin, norepinephrine and L-dopamine. Serotonin is involved with a number of behavioral functions in your body including the full feeling you experience after a meal. Additionally, serotonin affects your mood. A 1990 study found that women on conventional low calorie diets experienced clinical depression. A 1985 study commented that certain behaviors including preoccupation with food, were also prevalent in patients on low calorie diets that were also low in protein.

Dieting is only a temporary solution. You must adjust your eating patterns to reflect permanent changes that you know you are able to maintain forever. In other words, you must eat the same way while you are losing weight as you intend to eat once you have reached your ideal goal. Temporary food changes only mean temporary results. You do not need to deprive yourself, you just need to take control.

Speak with your doctor to help you determine your ideal weight. It will make it much easier for you to obtain the healthy results you are looking for.

## WHAT YOU EAT AFFECTS YOUR HEALTH

We have covered a lot of information so far and I want to be sure that you are not reading through the large lists of "what can happen if..." conditions and diseases and assume that you are not a likely candidate for any of them. Once again, disease and illness starts with what you put in your body. They don't attack you from out of nowhere. There is a reason that Americans have never been less healthy. As a society, we are more medicated now than we have ever been. Think about it... can you name ANYONE you know that is not taking some kind of medication for something? As a society, we are growing diseases within our bodies and are passing those diseases, often undetected, on to our offspring. In June of 2003, the Center For Disease Control warned that one in three children born in the year 2000 will become diabetic unless eating patterns are drastically changed.

During my tenure in the weight loss industry, I have had an opportunity to work with several blood labs that test blood to help people identify nutritional deficiencies. The reason that we have recommended they do that is because, in most cases, these people are experiencing symptoms or problems that usually have a deficiency base. I want to give you a list of physical conditions, many of which you may be experiencing, and let you know what can cause these problems and what nutrients you can take, either through food or through vitamin supplementation, to help eliminate them.

## I'll Start With The Most Common Deficiencies:

| SYMPTOM | CAUSE OR CONTRIBUTOR | NUTRIENT DEFICIENCY |
|---|---|---|
| Decreased learning capacity, age-related cognitive decline, Alzheimer's, fatigue, reduced endurance | Cooking & food processing, coffee, tea, alcohol Chronic dieting, drugs: antibiotics, diuretics, Phenytoin. | B 1 - Thiamine |
| Cracking, scaling skin; digestive abnormalities, mental confusion, anxiety, fatigue | High sugar consumption, low fat dieting, drugs: antibiotics | B 3 - Niacin |
| Depression, sleep problems, skin abnormalities, increased response to hypoglycemia, heart disease dementia, elevated homocysteine | Cooking & food processing, rancid fats in fried foods, alcohol, tobacco, soft drinks, bran. Drugs: antibiotics, estrogens, diuretics, oral contraceptives, theophylline | B2 deficiency B 6 - Pyridoxine |
| Anemia, impaired immune function, fatigue, Insomnia, premature hair loss, dysplasia, Birth defects, spinal bifida, certain cancers | Food processing/ cooking. Poor diet, advanced age drugs: aspirin, barbiturates, H2 blockers, steroids, oral contraceptives, valproic acid, phenytoin | Folic acid |
| Anemia, impaired immune function, mental deterioration, sleep disorders, fatigue, reduced Endurance. Elevated homocysteine, heart disease, dementia | Overgrown intestinal bacteria & parasites, stress alcohol, tobacco, caffeine, vegetarian diet drugs: antibiotics, H2 blockers, metaformin, proton pump inhibitors, potassium supplements | B 12 - Cyanoco- Balamin |
| Osteoporosis, osteomalacia, muscle cramping Irritability, acute anxiety, HTN, colon cancer, intestinal inflammation | High phosphorus foods (soft drinks, animal protein) excess dietary fiber. Drugs: aluminum hydroxide, barbiturates, antibiotics, steroids, digoxin and magnesium deficiency | Calcium |

| SYMPTOM | CAUSE OR CONTRIBUTOR | NUTRIENT DEFICIENCY |
|---|---|---|
| Muscle weakness/tremors, leg cramps, insomnia irregular heart rate, cardiac muscle spasm, anxiety, fatigue, depression, confusion, increased allergic responses | Soil depletion/food growth, excess calcium intake alcohol abuse, liver/kidney disease, diabetes, stress drugs: diuretics, steroids, estrogens, tetracyclines | Magnesium |
| Cancer, cataracts, macular degeneration, impaired immune function & toxin elimination atherosclerosis, elevated homocysteine | Disease, stress, protein deficient diet | N-acetyl cycteine and Glutathione |
| Cancer, cataracts, macular degeneration, wrinkled skin, arthrosclerosis, cancers | Disease, stress, poor diet barbiturates, antibiotics, steroids, digoxin and magnesium deficiency | Antioxidants |

### The following are less common or rare:

| | | |
|---|---|---|
| Anemia, cataracts, impaired thyroid function, fatigue, reduced endurance, elevated homocysteine, atherosclerosis | Poor diet. Drugs: antibiotics, tricyclic, oral Contraceptives, antidepressants | B 12- Riboflavin |
| Reduced stress tolerance, poor wound healing, skin problems, fatigue, reduced endurance | Alcohol, coffee & tea, smoking | B 5 - Pantothenic acid |
| Depression, nervous system abnormalities, wrinkles premature graying & hair loss, dry, scaly, skin, dementia, anxiety, depression, increased body fat, weight gain | Drugs: antibiotics, phynytoin, carbamazepine, diabetes low fat diet, poor dietary habits | Biotin Choline |
| Impaired immune function, poor wound healing, depression, impaired smell/taste; joint pain, skin, hair, nail problems. Fatigue, low endurance | Soil depletion/food prep. Protein/calorie restricted diet, alcoholism, diabetes, Drugs: ACE inhibitors Steroids, diuretics, H2 blockers, zidovudine | Zinc |
| Intestinal permeability to allergens/toxins; Food allergies, inflammatory arthritis, fatigue, skin eruptions, impaired immune function, poor wound healing | Disease, stress, poor diet | Glutamine |

As you can see from these charts, ailments that you may be experiencing can be treated and even cured by taking the proper nutrients. It makes sense that a diet deficient in calcium will cause the body to experience osteoporosis. Doesn't it make more sense to eat calcium-rich foods to ward off and avoid osteoporosis rather than wait until you are inflicted with the disease, then take prescription medicines to treat its affects?

When you review a chart such as this, we hope you realize the impact proper nutrition has toward fighting disease. In many instances, you will notice that prescription and over-the-counter drugs are often the culprit contributing to physical abnormalities. It is interesting to note that, for every $1.00 spent on prescription drugs, an additional $1.00 is spent on its adverse effects and treating the problems that drug has caused. Drugs are generally prescribed to treat symptoms and rarely treat the cause of most health problems. As consumers, the American public has learned to treat prescriptions as though they were magic solutions to life-threatening conditions. We cannot tell you how many people we have worked with that have taken cholesterol medications while continuing to eat high-cholesterol foods. They felt the medication was their protection against health issues associated with their poor food choices.

# HORMONE ENHANCING FOODS

From age twenty throughout the thirties, hormones begin to decrease. People who "eat whatever they want and never have a weight problem", suddenly get a dose of reality by age thirty and usually find themselves gaining unwanted pounds and inches. A hormone decrease sets your body up for metabolic problems.

There are foods you can eat to enhance your natural hormones. Even if you are taking prescription hormone medications, like Synthroid or Premarin, eating properly can only improve your hormone balance. The most critical hormones to balance for weight loss are thyroid, insulin, glucagon, and cortisol. We will also address growth hormone, testosterone, estrogen and progesterone because these hormones affect how your body ages and are greatly influenced by the "weight loss" hormones.

**Insulin, Glucagons and Cortisol.** These have been addressed at great length in the *Insulin* portion of this book. Avoiding sugars and starchy carbohydrates are required for good hormone health. Proteins and vegetables are the most important food categories to maintain proper balance of these hormones and should be the mainstay of your daily eating plan.

**Thyroid:** The most critical hormone for overall metabolism, thyroid controls the metabolism in every cell in your body. It also allows all other hormones to work properly. If your thyroid production is low, all other hormones are affected. Thyroid is the exception to the rule of low carbohydrate eating. To help the conversion of T4 to T3, (thyroid indicators), you need to eat complex carbohydrates. However, moderate amounts will suffice. In addition, carbs should only be eaten in the morning because that is when thyroid output is greatest.

**Foods To Increase Thyroid Production:**
- High protein, preferably organic foods such as free-range cattle and fish from unpolluted waters or deep seas
- Specific fruits provide good nutrients for your thyroid, but use sparingly due to their high sugar content (follow food guide):
  - Bananas
  - Grapefruits
  - Pineapple
  - Watermelon

- Mango
- Apples

▾ Brown rice, as a complex carbohydrate, is beneficial for thyroid function. Timing for eating these carbs is crucial. Ideally, they should only be eaten in the morning, before noon, and avoided for the rest of the day.

▾ Green leafy vegetables such as spinach and kale  *

▾ Tyrosine, which comes from protein sources and whey

**\* Food preparation is also important**. Some foods can interfere with the thyroid if cooked. Cooking destroys the blocking compounds in these otherwise nutritious foods:

- Broccoli
- Brussel sprouts
- Turnips
- Mustard greens
- Rutabaga

**Key Thyroid-Enhancing Supplements:** Vitamin A, C, E, B-Complex, Bioflavinoids which complement the B's, grape seed extract and quercitin; Minerals: Selenium, zinc, copper, chromium, manganese, magnesium, kelp and seaweed, which are rich in iodine and boosts thyroid function.

**Foods That Hinder Thyroid Production And Should Be Avoided:**

▾ Sugar

▾ Alcohol

▾ Caffeine

▾ Tobacco

▾ Milk has a thyroid-lowering protein.

▾ These foods can block the thyroid if taken in large amounts:
- Walnuts
- Sorghum
- Millet
- Tapioca

- Soy, in excessive quantities, contains a substance called genistein which can block the production of thyroid hormone.
- Nitrates interfere with the production of thyroid hormone and are prominent in the following foods: hot dogs, salami, deli meats
- Flouride, in toothpaste, water, or supplements, is a very potent thyroid disruptor.

**Adrenal And Sex Hormones: Estrogen, Progesterone, Testosterone, DHEA**
All of these adrenal and sex hormones are present in both males and females. The important relationship is the ratio of each hormone to each other. This ratio is what determines body fat, body shape, and metabolism. Production of all these hormones requires animal protein and good fats. Many studies have shown that vegetarians or people on extremely low fat diets, (which have been recommended for the past twenty years) have low androgens and sex hormones. Other studies show that people on low protein diets have low testosterone and low muscle mass. To produce all the adrenal and sex hormones required, the body needs adequate protein from meat, fish, chicken or eggs. It also needs adequate fat because all of these hormones are made from cholesterol. If cholesterol is too low, which can be as a result of cholesterol-lowering drugs or an extremely low fat diet, these important hormones will be low causing the endocrine system to be out of balance.

**Foods To Increase Adrenal & Sex Hormone Production:**
- Animal proteins
- Healthy, essential fatty acid foods like fish and avocado
- Spicy and salty foods

**Special note for men:** Sugar and beer increases estrogen. This causes a man to have a "beer belly" and women-like breasts. High estrogen production is bad in men and acts against testosterone.

**Testosterone:**  High insulin is the biggest offender and pushes down testosterone levels.

### Best Foods To Eat For Increased Testosterone Production:
- Protein (meat, fish, poultry and eggs.)
- Saturated fats like butter
- Monounsaturated oils such as olive oil, avocado oil and walnut oil.

### Foods That Hinder Testosterone Production And Should Be Avoided:
- Caffeine
- Alcohol
- Sugar
- All insulin-raising foods.

**Growth Hormone:**  The combination of amino acids in protein both stimulate increased growth hormone production and also increases the potency of your natural growth hormone by providing the amino acid building blocks necessary to build lean muscle, bones, skin, and hair. Growth Hormone is what makes you look younger and more vibrant.

### Best Foods To Eat For Increased Growth Hormone Production:
- Eat lots of protein, especially meat
- fish
- poultry
- eggs

### Foods That Hinder Growth Hormone Production And Should Be Avoided:
- Alcohol
- Coffee
- Sugar and carbohydrates

**Key Growth Hormone-Enhancing Supplements:**  Nutrients especially beneficial are arginine (4 grams at bedtime) and glutamine (2 grams at bedtime).

The more you know about yourself and the health of your parents and grandparents, the better you will be able to systematically direct your behavioral changes. Be honest. One USDA study revealed that more than 80% of the women who participated underestimated their daily food intake by more than 700 calories! In this instance, you have no one to fool but yourself.

## WEIGHT HISTORY

How much weight would you like to lose? _____ lbs.

Current weight _____ lbs          Goal weight _____ lbs.

How long have you been overweight? _____ years _____ Most of my life

How often do you weigh yourself?   0 Daily 0 Weekly 0 Monthly 0 Never

Why do you want to lose weight? (You may indicate as many as apply to you.)

0 Health      0 Appearance      0 Event      0 Family pressure      0 Doctor

What weight loss programs have you tried in the past.

0 Jenny Craig _____         0 Nutri-Systems _____         0 LA Weight Loss _____
0 Metabolife _____          0 Stacker      _____          0 Weight Watchers _____
0 Phen Fen / Redux _____    0 Other _____             0 South Beach _____

How much weight did you lose with them?   _____ lbs.

Did the weight stay off?          Yes          No Some

Why did you stop the program?    0 Too complicated    0 Too expensive
   0 Stopped working             0 Didn't like the food   0 Got boring

**Why do you think you have a weight problem?**    (Indicate as many as apply to you.)

0 Eat too much     0 Don't exercise    0 Eat wrong things     0 Dine out a lot
0 Family pressures 0 Stress eater      0 Overweight parents   0 Snacker
0 Eat too little   0 Travel            0 Demanding schedule   0 Don't know

**What keeps you motivated to stay on a program?** (Indicate as many as apply to you.)

0 Program support  0 Family support  0 Regular communication
0 Results          0 Strict guidelines 0 Planned meals
0 Minimal restrictions            0 Simplicity
0 Other: _____

## EATING HABITS

**How would you describe your eating?** (Select one from each line)

0 Picky Eater    0 Small Eater    0 Medium Eater    0 Large Eater
0 Healthy        0 Average        0 Fast food       0 Poor

Where do you usually eat?

0 Home        0 Dine out        0 Take lunch        0 Fast food

How many times per week do you eat out?  _____ times

How many dinners per week do you eat at home?_____ dinners at home

How often do you eat fast food?  _____ meals per week

Do you eat Breakfast?
0 Every day        0 Most days        0 Some days        0 Essentially never

Lunch?
0 Every day        0 Most days        0 Some days        0 Essentially never

Dinner?
0 Every day        0 Most days        0 Some days        0 Essentially never

What is your largest meal of the day?
0 Breakfast        0 Lunch        0 Dinner

**What do you consider your problem food areas:** (Indicate as many as apply to you.)

| | | | |
|---|---|---|---|
| 0 Starches (bread, pasta) | 0 Sweets | 0 Desserts | 0 Snacking |
| 0 Fast Food | 0 Skip meals | 0 Chips | 0 Cheese |

Do you tend to eat the same foods most of the time?   Yes    No    Sometimes

Do you cook?    0 Every day       0 Most days       0 Some days
                      0 Essentially never

Do you eat snacks? 0 Every day      0 Most days       0 Some days
                      0 Essentially never

**What snacks do you prefer?** (Indicate as many as apply to you.)

| | | | |
|---|---|---|---|
| 0 Ice Cream | 0 Cheese | 0 Chips | 0 Candy |
| 0 Chocolate | 0 Leftovers | 0 Fruit | 0 Protein bars |
| 0 protein shakes | | 0 Cereal | 0 Other |

What hours do you snack most?
   0 Early AM       0 Mid-day       0 Early Eve       0 Late PM

Do you consider yourself a stress or emotional eater?  Yes    No    Sometimes

**What foods do you like?** (Indicate as many as apply to you.)

| | | | |
|---|---|---|---|
| Red meat | Yes No | How often? | _____ times per week |
| Chicken | Yes No | | _____ times per week |
| Turkey | Yes No | | _____ times per week |
| Fish | Yes No | | _____ times per week |
| Pork | Yes No | | _____ times per wee |
| Veal | Yes No | | _____ times per week |
| Sausage | Yes No | | _____ times per week |
| Bacon | Yes No | | _____ times per week |
| Fruit | Yes No | | _____ times per week |
| Vegetables | Yes No | | _____ times per week |
| Bread | Yes No | | _____ times per week |
| Potato/Rice | Yes No | | _____ times per week |

| Pasta | Yes No | How often? | _____ times per week |
| Dairy/yogurt | Yes No | | _____ times per week |

Do you prefer:
  0 white bread      0 wheat bread      0 whole grain      0 rye
  0 white potato     0 sweet potato     0 fries
  0 white rice       0 brown rice       0 wild rice

What beverages do you usually drink?  (Indicate as many as apply to you.)
  0 Water      0 Coffee      0 Tea      0 Soda
  0 Juice      0 Wine        0 Beer     0 Cocktails

How many 8 oz. glasses of water do you drink daily?
  1            2            3            4            5+

How many cups of coffee do you drink daily?
  1         2         3         4            5            6+

What kind of coffee do you drink?
  0 Decaf      0 Regular      0 Cappuccino      0 Expresso

How often do you drink alcohol?
  0 Daily      0 Weekly      0 Monthly

How many glasses each occasion?
  1         2         3         4            5            6+

## LIFESTYLE

| | | | |
|---|---|---|---|
| Do you have a stressful job? | Ye | No | Sometimes |
| Do you have unusual hours? | Yes | No | Sometimes |
| Do work hours affect the times that you eat? | Yes | No | Sometimes |
| Are you stressed over your weight/health? | Yes | No | Sometimes |

Do you exercise?                                   Yes        No          Sometimes

How often?            _____ hours        _____ days per week

Where?
   0 Gym              0 Home              0 Classes          0 Bike
   0 Tennis           0 Golf              0 Walk             0 Yoga

Do you travel?        Yes                  No                  Sometimes
How Often? _____ days per month

Are you interested in nutrition?        Yes        No      Sometimes

Do you use the internet for information?  Yes        No      Sometimes

Have you told friends & family about your weight loss efforts?  Yes        No

Are they supportive?                                       Yes    No

Is your spouse overweight?                                 Yes    No

Are your children overweight?                              Yes    No

What is your favorite free time activity?   (Indicate as many as apply to you.)

   0 Reading           0 Relaxing          0 Golfing       0 Sewing
   0 Gardening         0 Tennis            0 Yoga
   0 Other       _____

Do you consider yourself in:

   0 Good health       0 Average Health  0 Poor Health

Do you feel your current weight is jeopardizing your health?   Yes        No

# MEDICAL HISTORY

We have also included a few charts that you may want to complete that will enable you to identify any patterns that may arise in your personal medical and family history. In this instance, what you are looking for is the identification of:

- Under-active thyroid
- Low growth hormone potential
- Low essential fatty acid content
- Toxins, candida, and allergies

If any of these conditions are part of your history, you may want to review the enclosed completed charts with your family doctor. Because thyroid problems can greatly restrict weight loss and health efforts, you may want to take the Barnes Temperature Test. Temperature is related to metabolic rate. Although it is not conclusive and should be confirmed by your doctor, if your basal temperature is low, it is a good indication that you may have a sluggish metabolism. This may also be related to low thyroid which is not always detected in traditional thyroid testing. Blood tests are notoriously inaccurate and many people who have "normal" thyroid blood tests are actually suffering from an under-active thyroid which will greatly affect their ability to lose weight.

The thyroid controls metabolism, the rate of burning fats, and body weight. Thyroid hormone acts on every cell in the body and enables all other hormones to work properly. Thyroid deficiencies interfere with the function of almost all bodily systems. A sluggish thyroid is probably the most undiagnosed cause of obesity and overweight. As we age, most of our hormones decline. Thyroid hormone allows the adrenal hormones to work efficiently, and vice versa, so it is important that the thyroid be operating properly. The same holds true for the gonadal and pituitary. They are all interconnected, essential and under the control of the master gland - the pituitary.

The brain and glandular system has extensive cross-communication between the thyroid, hypothalmus, adrenals and sex hormone system. The thyroid controls the rate of metabolism, thermogenesis and the burning of food, as well as enabling all cells in the body to burn sugar and fat optimally.

It is estimated that approximately 20% of the population with "normal" thyroid blood tests actually suffer from low thyroid function. Even if you do test "normal", you want to be at the upper 50% of the "normal" range, not at the bottom. Being at the bottom of a normal range will compromise your ability to lose weight. It will also contribute to continual weight fluctuations as well as cholesterol and heart challenges. Exercise will help boost metabolism so you don't always need medication if you are in the low-normal range. A simple basal temperature taken under the arm in the morning for four consecutive days will be a good indicator of thyroid health.

## THYROID: HOW TO TAKE THE BARNES TEST ●

**WOMEN:** This test should be done the first few days AFTER the beginning of your period. Women's basal temperatures vary throughout the month with their menstrual cycle. Post menopausal women may take it at any time.

**MEN:** Can be taken any time of the month.

### What To Do
Take your temperature before you get out of bed in the morning. Do not sit up. Prepare the mercury thermometer the night before and keep it within reach on a bedside table. Shake the mercury down thoroughly before you go to sleep. After waking in the morning, place the thermometer under your arm with your arm comfortably at your side. You should be reclined and relaxed. It is important that you do NOT get out of bed for any reason prior to or during the taking of this test. Stay in bed for about 10 minutes. Read and record the results. Follow this same instruction for 4-6 consecutive days.

If your temperature is consistently below 97.8 and you are complaining of any of the following symptoms, you may likely have a sluggish thyroid and should consult with your physician:

- Family history or thyroid problem
- Difficulty losing weight
- Dry, coarse hair
- Dry, scaly or rough skin
- Puffy face or bloating
- Fatigue, even after a night's sleep
- Cold intolerance
- Frequent headaches
- Infertility
- Slow heart rate
- Hypertension (high blood pressure)
- Depression
- Attention deficit disorder (ADD/ADHD)

* Weight gain and/or obesity
* Acne or rashes
* Hair loss
* Swelling of the feet or hands
* Constipation
* Chronic infection
* Joint and muscle pains
* Menstrual irregularity
* Shortness of breath
* High cholesterol
* Poor memory or concentration
* Anxiety and worry
* Chronic fatigue syndrome

## Family History

| Condition | Grandparents | Parents | Siblings | Children |
|---|---|---|---|---|
| Heart Disease/Bypass Surgery | | | | |
| High Blood Pressure | | | | |
| Diabetes | | | | |
| Obesity | | | | |
| Thinness | | | | |
| Skin Disorders (Psoriasis, Eczema, Acne) | | | | |
| Thyroid Disease | | | | |
| Stroke | | | | |
| Depression | | | | |

| Condition | Grandparents | Parents | Siblings | Children |
|---|---|---|---|---|
| Auto-Immune Disease | | | | |
| Arthritis | | | | |
| Crohn's Disease, Irritable Bowel | | | | |
| Allergies | | | | |
| Cancer | | | | |
| Early Death (under 50) | | | | |

| Hormones | Never | Sometimes | Often |
|---|---|---|---|
| 1. Sensitive to cold: General, feet, hands | | | |
| 2. Colder than other people in the room | | | |
| 3. fatigue, low energy, sleepy | | | |
| 4. tired when first wake up | | | |
| 5. swelling of the eyelids, hands and feet, and puffy face | | | |
| 6. constipated, bloated, slow digestion | | | |
| 7. dry, brittle hair and dry, rough skin | | | |
| 8. hair loss, hair thinner than it used to be | | | |
| 9. nails, brittle and slow-growing | | | |
| 10. weight gain | | | |

| Hormones | Never | Sometimes | Often |
| --- | --- | --- | --- |
| 11. depression, nervous, irritable, apathy | | | |
| 12. poor memory and poor concentration | | | |
| 13. joint and muscle cramps and stiffness | | | |
| 14. headaches, especially migraine | | | |
| 15. adult acne | | | |
| 16. poor thirst and poor sweating | | | |
| 17. irregular menstrual periods and severe PMS | | | |
| 18. Loss of muscle mass, weakness | | | |
| 19. Sagging jowls, turkey neck | | | |
| 20. hanging underarms, drooping inner thighs, sagging butt (poor muscle tone) | | | |
| 21. increased fat around abdomen | | | |
| 22. Fat pads above knees | | | |
| 23. Deeply wrinkled face, especially edge of eyes and mouth | | | |
| 24. Thin skin, thin hair, thin lips | | | |
| 25. Poorly muscled and wrinkled back of hands. | | | |
| 26. Loss of confidence, vitality, zest, not aggressive enough, low self-esteem, feels powerless | | | |

| Hormones | Never | Sometimes | Often |
|---|---|---|---|
| 27. Anxiety, depression, cannot tolerate stress, poor sleep | | | |
| 28. Dry, scaly, flaky skin | | | |
| 29. Dandruff | | | |
| 30. Pain and stiffness in joints | | | |
| 31. Dry, lackluster hair | | | |
| 32. Soft or brittle nails | | | |
| 33. Excessive thirst | | | |
| 34. Menstrual cramps | | | |

| TOXINS, CANDIDA, ALLERGY | Never | Sometimes | Often |
|---|---|---|---|
| 1. Dark circles under eyes or itching eyes | | | |
| 2. Skin itches or rashes for no apparent reason | | | |
| 3. Red, itchy rash of armpit, inner thigh or buttocks | | | |
| 4. Feel sleepy after meal | | | |
| 5. Bloated and distended belly, or gas after meal | | | |
| 6. Rashes or itching between toes or nail discoloration | | | |
| 7. Large mood and energy swings | | | |

| TOXINS, CANDIDA, ALLERGY | Never | Sometimes | Often |
|---|---|---|---|
| 8. Extremely sensitive to smells, perfumes, cleaning chemicals, cigarette smoke | | | |
| 9. Congestion or itching of nose, throat, ear, or sinuses, or cough | | | |
| 10. Travel outside the US | | | |
| 11. Received 2 courses of antibiotics within the past 5 years | | | |
| 12. Do you feel better or worse (circle) after antibiotics | | | |
| 13. Have more than 2 "silver" fillings in mouth | | | |
| 14. Lot of dental problems--gums, root canals, lost teeth | | | |
| 15. Headaches, migraines | | | |
| 16. Are you sensitive to molds, pets, dust, worse on muggy damp days or moldy places | | | |
| 17. Crave sugar or bread or specific food like chocolate | | | |
| 18. Eating specific food gives one pain, cramps, or diarrhea | | | |

**If you see patterns emerging, share these charts with your doctor.**

# THE BENEFITS OF EXERCISE ●

There is no question that we always feel better when we exercise and use our muscles. Recognize that it does not have to be painful or difficult in order to be effective.

Why exercise? Simple. You can eat more when you preserve muscle and lose fat. When dieting without exercise, you lose a combination of fat and muscle mass. 25% of all weight lost without exercise comes from muscle loss. **Muscle burns 40 calories per pound. Fat burns 2 calories per pound.** The heavier or higher your body fat content, the fewer calories you can eat every day just to maintain your current weight. If we can help you lose more fat and less muscle, or, better yet, build more muscle mass, you will be able to eat more and still maintain your ideal weight. Please be aware that your increased protein consumption will also help you accomplish this goal.

Aerobic activities benefit your cardiovascular system. The word 'aerobic' literally means with oxygen. When you do aerobic exercise, your goal is to maintain a consistent heart rate over a given period of time. Initially, you may not be able to keep your heart rate up for very long. Start slowly and build up. As you become more consistent with your exercise efforts, you will be surprised at how much more endurance you will achieve.

Weight training focuses more on muscle development than the heart. This is also a good option for those who prefer not to 'sweat' as much. Using weights will help you reshape your body, increase lean muscle and bone mass while making you stronger.

If you have done little or no exercise before, be careful not to over-train in your enthusiasm. Let your muscles rest every other day until you feel you can do more. Be sure to stretch real well before you begin any exercise.

In addition to the calorie and fat burning that exercise offers, it is also an excellent way to help prevent many diseases. Research shows that aerobic exercise reduces joint pain and arthritis symptoms. Exercise also helps with osteoporosis, hypertension, premenstrual tension and helps keep blood sugar levels in a normal range for diabetics. Cholesterol levels are also reduced.

It is also important for you to understand that exercise for weight loss is not necessarily required every day nor do you need to kill yourself to the point of exhaustion in the gym. Surprisingly enough, "less is more" when it comes to exercising for weight loss.

## You Have Two Options:

Ideally you should do a combination of both aerobic and anaerobic exercise. Each type has profound but different effects on your hormones which burn fat and shape your body.

**Aerobic exercises,** which are heart elevating exercises like treadmill, bike, spinning and Stairmaster, all burn fat. To maximize your aerobic workout, all that is required is to elevate your heart rate to a target range and maintain that rate for 20 minutes in order to burn the maximum amount of fat.

**To calculate the best weight loss heart range,** all you need to do is deduct your age from 220 then take 70-80% of that number. For example:

*If you were 45 years old:   220 - 45 = 175*
*70% of 175 = 123  /  80% of 175 = 140*

For maximum fat burn the example person above needs to keep their heart rate between 123 and 140 beats per minute. When your resting heart rate is between 80 & 90, it may not take much exercise to elevate it into this weight loss range. You may not even break a sweat yet your exercise effort will still be effective. In fact, experts tell us that if you elevate your heart too high, following the "no pain no gain" concept, it will be counter-productive when it comes to fat burn and weight management. When you do aerobic exercises, your body is using your fat storage for energy.

**Anaerobic exercises,** like resistance or weight training exercises, are designed to burn sugar while building muscle. In this instance, your body is burning glucose or sugar for energy, not fat. But, by maintaining or building muscle mass, your body is able to process more calories so you can eat more. Remember, muscle burns 40 calories per pound and fat burns only 2 calories per pound. Resistance training also tends to increase growth hormone, testosterone and glucagons more than aerobic exercise. That is why a balance of the two is recommended.

**Over-exercising,** or elevating your heart too much when doing aerobic exercises will actually put your body into an anaerobic state where it stops burning fat and starts burning muscle. Once you have reached this state, it is very difficult for your body to re-enter an aerobic state again. Once it starts burning muscle, it will continue to do so which means you will need to stop exercising and come back at least one hour later, or on another day.

**Heart Monitors give aerobic assurance** because they allow you to verify that you are keeping your heart rate within your personal fat-burning range. Heart rate monitors work for your body like a tachometer works for your car. It shows you how hard your engine is working.

**Why do I need anaerobic exercise too?** For long-term weight loss results, you need to lose fat while at least maintaining muscle. Aging causes us to lose muscle mass each year. If you don't work out to maintain or rebuild what you lose, every year you will need to eat less-and-less just to maintain your current weight.

**Hormone healthy exercise:** Exercise has a dramatic effect on your hormones and you need both aerobic and anaerobic exercise. The first for fat burning, and the second for muscle strength and growth. In order to exercise in a hormonally sensible way and maximize anabolic hormones, the best time is in the early morning when testosterone is high and insulin is low, so you will burn fat and not sugar. If you exercise later in the day when insulin is high, you will not be able to mobilize the fat you want to burn. In addition, and for exactly the same reason, exercise should be done on an empty stomach.

Exercise will stimulate growth hormone, testosterone and glucagon secretion. However, if done after a meal when insulin is high, then beneficial hormones will be suppressed and you will not burn fat. Instead, you will remain a "sugar burner" and possibly also release cortisol which will keep your sugar level up. When this happens, muscle tissue will begin to burn rapidly too.

**Walking is best.** Dr. Lewis recommends walking as the single best exercise. We all know how to do it, it is safe on the joints; it uses the largest weight bearing muscles, and stimulates anabolic hormones. As a cardiologist, he had 90% of his post-heart attack patients walking at least one mile per day just one month after their acute heart attack. The benefits were astounding. There is no reason why anybody cannot gradually build up their ability to walk one mile in twenty minutes if they are consistently walking over a period of one month.

If you have knee or hip problems, pool exercises, the Ellipser, or a stationary bicycle may be more comfortable. Remember, as you strengthen your thigh muscles, your knee problems may improve because the thigh muscles give stability to your knee.

Weight training has an even greater effect on hormone health because it increases growth hormone and testosterone even more than aerobic training. It helps build muscles, as well as preserve muscle tissue. As you lose weight, it even stimulates more fat burn.

All proper exercise burns food for energy and leads to increased nutritional demands for energy-promoting nutrients such as the B-vitamins, C, Manganese, Zinc, Magnesium and Selenium. It also requires an increased need for antioxidants such as vitamin A, C, E, MSM, NAC, Lycopene, Co-Q 10, Curcumin, in order to quell the increased free radical storm generated by exercise and the increased food metabolism it causes.

We cannot stress enough that the cardinal rule about all exercise is to take your time. You have years ahead of you to sculpt your body, there is no need to try to redesign it in a month. Go slowly and be safe. If you over-do your workout program and injure yourself, the result will most likely be no exercise program at all, which will cause your muscles to atrophy. Remember, muscle is your body's main source of energy and calorie burning. If you lose your muscle mass, your body's overall ability to burn food will slow dramatically and the excess, unused fuel will be stored as fat.

Be good to yourself and add exercise to help fulfill your daily balance in life. You can alternate between aerobic and weight training each day too. But, be consistent. Your body and your lifestyle will thank you for it.

# FOOD ALLERGIES ARE REAL & DANGEROUS  ●

Even when you follow all the rules, it is possible that your body will still fight weight loss. Although it's hard to deny the discouragement and frustration this situation causes, the fact is, we have already determined that you can't lose weight if your body won't let you. Food allergies and all they encompass will stop your body from operating properly too.

People have reactions to certain types of foods that are not related to the chemicals or fats those foods contain. Food allergies, intolerance's and sensitivities are three separate food reactions that may be very dangerous to your health, can affect weight loss or weight maintenance efforts, and may even cause death.

Unfortunately, some allergies or sensitivities are active without showing any symptoms. Indigestion, nausea, skin rashes, and sinus congestion can all be indications of food allergies. But, your inability to lose weight when you know you are doing everything right is another indication that sensitivities may be present. Even reactions to non-caloric items like onion or artificial sweeteners may cause your body to retain unwanted fat by metabolically slowing down. Simple food sensitivity tests can be performed by a family doctor. This test is highly recommended to help determine which foods should be avoided or, at least, minimized.

Most food allergy sufferers only experience temporary discomfort, however, many undiagnosed allergies can lead to chronic degenerative diseases. For those whose allergies are more acute, they may go into a type of shock or their throats can swell enough to cut off breathing. Although there are as many as two hundred food ingredients that can provoke food allergies, the vast majority of serious reactions are caused by only nine. They are:

| | |
|---|---|
| • Nuts | * Peanuts (which are legumes not nuts) |
| • Milk | * Eggs |
| • Fish | * Shellfish |
| • Strawberries | * Soybeans |
| • Wheat | |

Food intolerances like lactose intolerance, is not the same as an allergy. People who are lactose intolerant may only be susceptible to milk and can oftentimes continue to eat small amounts of dairy products like cheese, ice cream, and yogurt which contain much less lactose or can be purchased 'lactose free'. Each person has a different threshold as to how much lactose they can tolerate without symptoms.

It can be very difficult to identify food allergies without the help of your doctor. Many products contain ingredients which some people are unknowingly sensitive Progresso Chicken Noodle Soup, for example, is not just made with chicken & noodles. It contains soy, egg whites, and MSG - all potential food allergy triggers.

It is very important that you recognize how you feel after eating certain kinds of foods. If you experience discomfort after a meal, try to identify what you ate and see if you experience the same discomfort when you eat any of those same items again. Good health and weight management depends upon proper body balance. If you do not feel well or if you have stomach upset after eating, your body is trying to tell you that something is wrong. If specific foods cause you to feel poorly, those foods should be avoided. Another sign of a food allergy will be a significant increase in heart rate after eating the culprit food.

Product labels may not always provide you with the information you need if food allergies are present. They do not have to include known allergens within the label text if those ingredients are not in enough quantity to require disclosure. For example, when foods contain flavorings that come from plants or animals, the ingredient list need only say "natural flavor" even though those flavors may contain allergens from nuts, eggs or milk.

Be aware of your body and how it reacts to food. If you listen, your body will usually tell you just about everything you need to know in order to nutritionally fortify it properly. When allergic or intolerant foods are eliminated from your diet, weight loss is often rapid and spectacular. So, if you have reached a plateau or weight loss is slow, consider food allergy or sensitivity testing.

# SUGAR FEEDS CANCER & PREMATURE AGING ●

As tasty as sugar is, very little good comes from eating it. It is the biggest contributor to weight problems, is responsible for lines, wrinkles and dimples on your skin and cancer experts agree that glucose (sugar) is cancer's preferred growth fuel. Excess blood sugar can initiate yeast overgrowth, blood vessel deterioration, heart disease and other health conditions. It damages the immune system which can promote infections and cancer.

You can take a lot of responsibility for your health by eating right. For the cancer patients participating in a four-year study at the National Institute of Public Health and Environmental Protection, cancer risk more than doubled for those patients who had high intake of sugars. Sugar was also credited for higher breast cancer rates in women, particularly those over 65. As a side note, sugar and the increased consumption of carbohydrates is also credited for the alarming increase in diabetes nationally.

For the best "cancer prevention diet" it is recommended that you minimize refined sugar products, eat more vegetables and less fruit. Refined sugar products include the obvious sweet treats, but white starches like white bread, white rice, pasta and potatoes are all heavy glucose producers too. These are the same sugars that will ultimately turn to fat in your body if you're not active enough to burn off all the sugar-creating foods you eat daily. Remember, it takes 15 minutes of jogging just to burn off the glucose created from 1 slice of bread. How much starch are YOU eating everyday?

These are scary statistics, particularly if cancer runs in your family. Protect yourself and focus on cancer fighting foods that are high in antioxidants. Here are a few suggestions:

**Eat whole grains whenever possible.** The darker and heavier the bread, the better it will be for you. Grains lessen colon cancer. But, remember, grains do eventually break down into sugar so eat them sparingly.

**Tea leaves** contain antioxidants called polyhpenols, which can prevent damage to DNA. If cells do turn cancerous, one group of polyphenols, called catechins, seems to prevent them from multiplying. Best bets: green or black tea, but not herbal teas. Water should be hot but not boiling.

**Tomatoes, red peppers, carrots, & strawberries** all have cancer fighting properties.

**Licorice root.** Best bet: get dried licorice root from local health food store and use as a stir-stick in tea. Special note: licorice candy is not made with licorice root.

**Oranges & lemons** both contain a substance that raises levels of naturally occurring enzymes thought to break down carcinogens and stimulate cancer-killing cells. Other good bets: Limes and other citrus fruits, as well as cardamom, celery and the seeds of caraway and fennel.

**Grapes** are loaded with ellagic acid, which blocks the body's production of enzymes used by cancer cells. In a few cancer studies, concord grapes were as effective as the cancer drug methotrexate in slowing tumor growth.

**Garlic & onions.** A study of 41,000 women in Iowa showed that those who added garlic to their menu at least once a week reduced their risk of colon cancer by 35%. Onions also increase levels of enzymes that break down potential carcinogens. Scallions and chives also fall into this category.

**Chile peppers**. The hotter the pepper, the more effective it will be.

**Soybeans.** Rich in genistein, this chemical found in soybeans may fight cancer cells in the breast and ovaries. Other good bets: Tofu, soy milk, soy flour, miso, mung beans and alfalfa sprouts.

**Broccoli & cabbage, brussels sprouts, cauliflower, bok choy, kale, mustard seed & radishes** all contain beta carotene, and are powerful, natural cancer fighters.

## *Other Cancer-Fighters*

The following is a list of cancer-fighting tips developed by the nation's leading food scientists.  Here's what you can do to lower your cancer risk:

▽ **Don't smoke or use smokeless tobacco** - decreases lung, pancreas, stomach, bladder, esophagus, mouth and throat cancer.

▽ **If you drink alcoholic beverages,** limit them to 1 drink per day for women and 2 per day for men - this will lesson breast, liver, esophagus, mouth and throat cancers.

▽ **Cut back on 'bad' fats** - lessen colon, breast, prostate, pancreas and ovarian cancer.

▽ **Eat whole grains or high fiber foods whenever possible** - lessen colon cancer.

▽ **Exercise 3-4 hours a week** -  lessen colon and breast cancer.

▽ **Take an aspirin each day** (Check with doctor) - lessen colon cancer.

▽ **Limit or avoid cured or smoked meats like bacon, ham, lox & hotdogs.** If you must eat these items,  eat them with a glass of orange juice or another rich source of vitamin C to lessen potential for stomach cancer.

▽ **Limit salt consumption to 2400mg. or less daily** - lessen stomach cancer

▽ **Avoid obesity -** lessen breast, endometrium and numerous other cancers.

▽ **Eat at least 5-9 servings of fruits & vegetables daily -** lessen lung, colon, pancreas, stomach, bladder, esophagus, mouth and throat cancer.

# FOODS FOR YOUR FACE

Nutrition is just as important for your face as it is for your body. It is well documented that vitamin deficiencies lead to dry, flaky skin, hair loss, and brittle nails. Iron deficiency which is common among women of childbearing age, can leave complexions pale and drawn. Zinc shortages can cause flaky and rash-prone skin. Supplements can be part of the solution if regular, balanced meals are difficult. Here are a few skin essential foods and the role they play to help keep you fit.

**BETA-CAROTENE.** Sources: orange colored vegetables and fruits like carrots, sweet potatoes, squash, cantaloupe, apricots and spinach can improve skin cells.
*BENEFIT:* Considered to help ward off cancer.

**BIOTIN.** Sources: Cheese, eggs, peanut butter.
*BENEFIT:* Essential for strong hair and nails.

**ESSENTIAL FATTY ACIDS.** Sources: Cooking oils like corn, olive, safflower, fish, omega 3 fatty acids.
*BENEFIT:* Keeps skin moist and supple.

**IRON.** Sources: Red meat, broccoli, spinach.
*BENEFIT:* Deficiency can cause itchy, pale skin and fatigue.

**SELENIUM.** Sources: Meat, seafood, milk, vegetables, whole grains, walnuts.
*BENEFIT:* May reduce sun damage and protect against non-melanoma skin cancers.

**VITAMIN A.** Sources: Eggs, butter, liver.
*BENEFIT:* High doses have helped prevent recurrences of skin cancer. Deficiency can cause dry, flaky skin.

## HOW TO MAKE A VALUABLE SALAD ●

Unfortunately, salad, which is a staple for most women and is eaten as a meal for many, has little or no nutritional value. Most lettuce offers only minuscule amounts of fiber, folic acid and vitamins A and C while the dressing adds lots of fat. Iceberg lettuce, which is the one most used, actually has the lowest nutritional value of all.

If salad is going to continue to be an important part of your menu planning, make its food value higher by selecting the right greens and adding toppings with some nutritional value of their own. By mixing a variety of greens and vegetables, you'll not only be doing your body a favor, you'll provide more interest for your taste buds. Whatever salad you create, if it is to be eaten as a meal, be sure it includes a full serving (minimum 6-8 ounces) of protein like grilled chicken, beef, salmon, tuna or tofu.

| Greens in Order of Highest Food Value | Toppings With Vitamins & Fiber |
|---|---|
| Dandelion Greens | Alfalfa Sprouts |
| Garden Cress | Black beans, garbanzo, kidney |
| Kale & Spinach | Carrots |
| Watercress | Cabbage |
| Mustard Greens | Seeds - sesame, sunflower poppy |
| Swiss Chard | Nuts - Almonds, pignoli |
| Chicory | Fruit |
| Romaine | Avocado |
| Arugula | Cucumber |
| Endive | Tomatoes |
| Leaf - Green or Red | Cauliflower |
| Iceberg | Onion, scallions or chives |

Whenever possible, make your own dressing. Vinaigrette is lighter, has less fat and can have more flavor than creamy dressings. Mix 1/3 extra-virgin olive oil and 2/3 your favorite vinegar. Many balsamic vinegars have so much flavor, you don't even need oil. If they are too strong, you can effectively cut some of the flavor with water. For additional taste, include spices like oregano, garlic, lemon and pepper. When the contents of your salad have lots of flavor, heavy dressings are not as important.

# 8 MOST IMPORTANT NUTRIENTS FOR MEN

Men and women have different nutritional requirements. In fact, the US Food & Drug Administration puts out separate men's and women's lists of Recommended Dietary Allowances (RDA) for vitamins and minerals, although they usually use the 'men's' statistics when printing nutritional information on product supplement panels. Generally, men need more of just about every nutrient simply because they are usually bigger in size. However, men are especially high risk for health problems such as elevated cholesterol, hypertension, coronary heart disease, stroke, certain cancers and kidney stones. Getting the proper balance of vitamins and minerals will help fight against these health hazards.

### *Here is a list of the nutrients men need most and where to find them:*

**CHROMIUM.** The average man needs at least 50 micrograms of chromium a day, but you may have a hard time getting that much from foods. Wheat germ and American cheese are high in chromium but are not usually on your daily menu so take a multivitamin-mineral complex that includes chromium.

**FIBER.** Technically not a nutrient, fiber is known to reduce cholesterol, lower your risk of colon cancer, (the second most deadly kind for men), and control sugar levels in diabetics.

**MAGNESIUM.** This mineral plays a key role in regulating the heartbeat. Food sources are baked potato, beans, nuts, oatmeal, peanut butter, whole-wheat spaghetti, deep green leafy vegetables and seafood.

**VITAMIN B-6.** This necessary nutrient is a powerful immune booster and protects against the formation of kidney stones, which is a problem that afflicts twice as many men as women. It can also help prevent restless sleep. A man's daily requirement of two milligrams is about the amount found in two large bananas. Additional sources are chicken, fish, liver, rice, avocados, walnuts, wheat germ and sunflower seeds.

**VITAMIN C.** This vitamin boosts immunity, prevents cancer, heart disease and stroke. It also promotes healthy gums & teeth, prevents cataracts, hastens wound healing, counteracts asthma, helps ward off the common cold and may help over-come infertility. Your best sources are broccoli, orange juice, green peppers, strawberries and papayas. If you smoke, you probably need extra vitamin C.

**VITAMIN E.** This vitamin may lower cholesterol, prevent buildup of artery-clogging plaque, boosts immunity, cleanses the body of pollutants and prevents cataracts. There is a lot of 'E' in almonds, peanuts, pecans, wheat germ and canola oil.

**WATER.** Still the most important nutrient for your body. Eight, 8-ounce glass-es are required daily and, if you exercise regularly, double that amount. In fact, it is best if you drink half your body weight in ounces of water every day.

**ZINC.** Getting enough zinc may ensure your sex drive, potency and fertility for staying in shape. Men tend to get only 2/3 of the RDA of 15 milligrams. That is mostly because when men sweat, they lose more zinc than women do. One 4-ounce helping of lean beef provides almost half the daily zinc requirement. Other sources are turkey, oysters, cereals and beans.

# UNCORK THE FACTS ABOUT ALCOHOL ●

As we tip a few toddies at day's end, it's important to note the effect alcohol has on your body. Not only will drinking add it's own amount of calories to your daily total, researchers have found that the consumption of alcohol doesn't reduce the appetite - it stimulates it! That's right. Studies have shown that people who ate meals and drank alcoholic beverages consumed more food per meal than they did eating the same foods with non-alcoholic drinks.

The good news is, moderate drinking of red wine can actually help protect against heart disease. Moderate drinking means a maximum of two drinks per day although that number does not take exceptions into consideration. Two drinks per day is usually not appropriate for many women's chemistry, the elderly, or people taking prescription drugs.

It is true that studies have shown alcohol seems to raise the risk of breast cancer in women by raising levels of the hormone estrogen, which promotes the development of certain types of breast tumors. A Harvard study of almost 90,000 middle-aged women partaking in 3-9 drinks a week reduced the risk of heart disease by 40% but raised the risk of breast cancer by 30%. Even though these numbers may seem like a wash, the significant fact is that only 4% of all women die of breast cancer whereas 40% of women die of heart disease. This would mean that moderate drinking would actually extend more lives than it would end prematurely. However, this should not be your motivation to start drinking if you do not drink alcoholic beverages currently. If you're taking any medications, check with your doctor to see how alcohol will effect them.

Be smart. Even though some alcoholic beverages can improve health, remember that the alcohol content in drinks depresses or further slows what may be an already slow metabolism which will lessen your weight loss success. Enjoy your cocktails in moderation.

# NOW... TAKE CHARGE!

A little information goes a long way. Change is never easy but you will soon find that it is going to get increasingly difficult for you to enjoy French fries or other unhealthy foods when you consider all the terrible things that food is physically doing to you. Instant gratification becomes over-ruled by an increased desire to look and feel good. When you are tuned into your body, you will begin to recognize what foods make you feel great and which ones make you feel funky. Good health isn't out of your hands. Only you can be responsible for what you choose to put in your mouth or how much activity you'll make time for. It is simply a matter of priorities.

We often hear that "It's expensive to eat right... healthy food costs a lot more money." Depending upon the procedure, heart surgery costs well over $50,000.00. You can buy a lot of chicken, apples and vitamins with that kind of budget! Besides, there is nothing more expensive than packaged foods.

It's now up to you. You need to evaluate your life, what you know are the problem areas that require change, and what changes you are willing to make. It must come from you. In order to make any effective alteration or adjustment to diet or lifestyle, you must prefer and embrace the changes. Otherwise, you will eventually go back to the bad habits that you were desirous of breaking. Don't make it complicated. Make it real. You can do anything you set your mind to doing. So, what'll it be?

## ABOUT THE AUTHORS

*Debi Davis, BioDieteticsFounder*

Ms. Davis, along with her former husband, Byron, founded Fit America in 1991. Having personally lost 85 pounds and helping hundreds of thousands of others to do the same, Ms. Davis is viewed as an industry expert for practical and realistic weight loss practices. She has appeared in magazines such as Redbook, Fortune Small Business, Success, Newsweek, Entrepreneur, and more; is regularly interviewed by TV and news media such as CNN, Fox, ABC, NBC, USA Today and was Ernst & Young's 1999 Entrepreneur of the Year for health. Ms. Davis is a regular speaker and a published author of several books; "Weight Loss Through Visualization" and "Back Off! I'll Lose Weight When I'm Ready" and is a regular contributor to many books and periodicals such as Balance Magazine. In 2002, Ms. Davis, along with her partner and ex-husband, Byron, started Fit America M.D., a physician-led, medical partnering company that helps physicians throughout the United States help patients lose weight and get healthy through proper nutrition, lifestyle and exercise. That effort has now led the Davis' to develop a more sophisticated and medically-based consumer weight loss company, BioDietetics. Their commitment to the health of America is provided through personal coaching via their retail locations, website or toll-free number.

*Sylvan R. Lewis, M.D.*

Dr. Lewis created *The 7-Day Prep for Hormone Balance,* recognizing the association between proper hormone balance and weight reduction, it is the culmination of his thirty years as a practicing physician utilizing his diverse expertise in medicine and nutrition. He attended Columbia College, New York, and New York University Medical School where he graduated with honors and was recognized as one of the top 10% of America's medical school graduates. He is Board Certified in Internal Medicine and Cardiovascular Diseases and has a doctorate in Integrative Medicine. Dr. Lewis was Health and Nutrition Advisor to the U.S. Department of Health, Education and Welfare, and Chief of Cardiology at the U.S. Public Health Service Hospital in New Orleans, LA., where he served as Lt. Commander in the Navy. Dr. Lewis has been practicing medicine for over thirty years and has been a member of the staff of Parkway General Hospital, Aventura

Medical Center, and Mt. Sinai Hospital in Miami, Florida. He has published four books on nutrition and weight management: "Lose Ugly Fat Fast", "Dr. Lewis' Carbohydrate and Sugar Diet Guide", "Heart Watchers Complete Diet & Menu Planner" and "Diet & Exercise Made Easy". Recognizing the relationship between nutrition and physical health, Dr. Lewis is an honored leader in the health and wellness field.

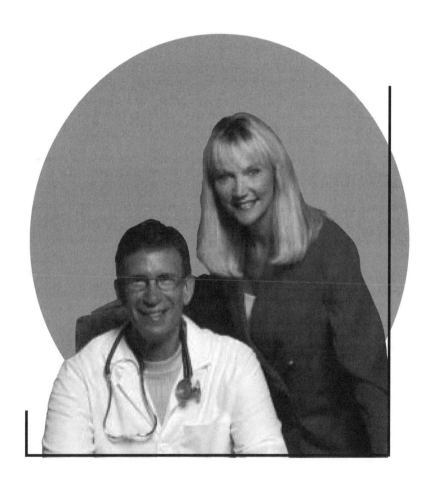

Shelbyville-Shelby County
Public Library